Measurement of Nursing Outcomes

Second Edition

Volume 3:
Self Care and Coping

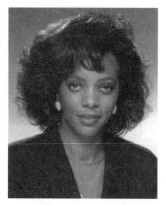

Ora L. Strickland, PhD, RN, FAAN, is a Research Scientist at the Atlanta Veterans Administration Medical Center and is professor in the Nell Hodgson Woodruff School of Nursing at Emory University in Atlanta, Georgia. She earned a doctoral degree in child development and family relations from the University of North Carolina, Greensboro; a master's degree in maternal and child health nursing from Boston University, Massachusetts; and a bachelor's degree in nursing from North Carolina Agricultural and Technical State University, Greensboro. Dr. Strickland coedited the original four volumes of *Measurement of Nursing Outcomes*. She is the founder and senior editor of the *Journal of Nursing Measurement*. An internationally known specialist in nursing research, measurement, evaluation, maternal and child health, and parenting. Dr. Strickland has published widely in professional journals and is frequently called upon as a consultant by health care agencies, universities, government agencies, and community organizations. She has presented more than 200 public lectures, speeches, and workshops, and her research has been featured in newspapers and magazines, as well as on radio and television.

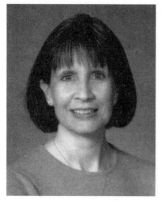

Colleen DiIorio, PhD, RN, FAAN, is a professor in the Department of Behavioral Sciences and Health Education at Rollins School of Public Health, Emory University and the Department of Family and Community Nursing in the Nell Hodgson Woodruff School of Nursing at Emory University. Dr. DiIorio earned a doctoral degree in nursing research and theory development from New York University. She received her master's degree in nursing, with a functional minor in delivery of nursing services, from New York University and received a bachelor's degree in nursing from the University of Iowa. Dr. DiIorio has extensive experience in health promotion research. She currently serves as principal investigator on four NIH-funded research grants. Her work covers two broad areas addressing health behavior and behavioral change: adherence/self-management and HIV prevention. Dr. DiIorio has published numerous articles and chapters on self-management and HIV prevention in addition to topics on measurement, health promotion, disease prevention, and evaluation. Dr. DiIorio has served as a consultant to and on panels of community organizations, governmental agencies, and professional organizations. She currently serves as associate editor of the *Journal of Nursing Measurement*.

Measurement of Nursing Outcomes

Second Edition

Volume 3:
Self Care and Coping

Ora Lea Strickland, PhD, RN, FAAN
Colleen Dilorio, PhD, RN, FAAN
Editors

 Springer Publishing Company

Springer Publishing Company, Inc.
536 Broadway
New York, NY 10012-3955

Acquisitions Editor: Ruth Chasek
Production Editor: Pam Lankas
Cover design by Joanne Honigman

03 04 05 06 07 / 5 4 3 2 1

Library of Congress Cataloging-in-Publication Data

Measurement of nursing outcomes / Ora L. Strickland, Colleen DiIorio, editors,— 2nd ed.
    p. cm.
    Includes bibliographical references and index.
    ISBN 0-8261-1795-3 (v. 3)
    1. Nursing—Standards. 2. Nursing audit. I. DiIorio, Colleen. II. Strickland, Ora L.
    [DNLM: 1. Nursing—methods. 2. Clinical Competence. 3. Nursing—standards. 4. Outcome and Process Assessment (Health Care). WY 16 M484 2001]
    RT85.5 .M434 2001
    610.73—dc21

                                     00-054928

Printed in the United States of America by Sheridan Books Inc.

CONTENTS

Preface

This volume of the *Measurement of Nursing Outcomes* book series provides nursing measurement tools that focus on self-care and coping. The new edition of this series updates and expands upon the original four volumes produced in 1988 and 1990 that were coedited by Carolyn F. Waltz and Ora L. Strickland. The major purposes of this publication are to

1. Keep client-focused nursing instruments easily accessible to those who need to use them,
2. Update some of the instruments that appeared in the original volumes by providing additional psychometric information, and
3. Encourage the dissemination of other nursing measures that are useful to the practice of nurse clinicians and researchers.

Over the past 20 years, much progress has been made in nursing measurement. The first four volumes of the *Measurement of Nursing Outcomes* book series were a direct outgrowth of the Measurement of Clinical and Educational Nursing Outcomes Project, which was funded by the Division of Nursing, Special Projects Branch, Department of Health and Human Services Grant 1D10NU23085. Over 200 nurse educators and researchers sharpened their skills in nursing measurement through this project by developing or modifying, and testing tools to measure nursing outcome variables. The skills that these nurses garnered through this project not only have increased the number of quality nursing measures but have improved the quality of measurement content taught in nursing programs. Given the recent focus on evidenced-based outcomes, progress made in this area has had a significant impact on nursing practice, quality of care assessment, and knowledge development and scholarship in the field.

This publication serves as a distinct representation of the progress made in the advancement of nursing measurement during the past decade and ushers the field into the 21st century with more stellar measurement instruments that better quantify key concepts and constructs that are important to nursing practice and research. It is presented with the full recognition that nurses can only provide the best of care, conduct the most potent and influential research, and effectively expand its knowledge base when its approaches to quantifying nursing variables are dependable, that is, measure the phenomena of interest reliably and accurately. In

essence, consistent and appropriate application of measurement principles and practices, along with the development of sensitive and valid
measures, is crucial if the profession of nursing is to continue to advance
and impact patient care.

A variety of instruments that address concepts relevant to self-care and
coping are presented in this volume. Several of the measures have been
designed for use in specific diseases, such as epilepsy, cancer, and diabetes. Others can be used with clients in the general population or with
various health care conditions. In general, four topical areas are addressed
by the instruments in this volume: Self-Efficacy and Self-Care, Coping,
Social Support and Quality of Life, and Measuring Health Behaviors. It is
our hope that the dissemination of these measurement tools will not only
facilitate outcome assessment and knowledge development but encourage their use and their further development and testing, thereby, advancing the state of nursing measurement even further. Although we have
come a long way in nursing measurement, work in the area needs to
continue. The strides forward that we have made thus far do not negate
the fact that we still have far to go and much work to be done.

ORA LEA STRICKLAND, PHD, RN, FAAN
COLLEEN DIIORIO, PHD, RN, FAAN

Acknowledgment

The editors gratefully acknowledge Regina M. Daniel, Administrative Assistant in the Rollins School of Public Health at Emory University, who graciously contributed her time and management skills to ensure the completion of this book. Her commitment, perseverance, and talents were liberally shared during the development of this book. Thank you, Regina. You are greatly appreciated.

Contributors

Karen J. Aroian, PhD, RN, CS, FAAN
Katherine E. Faville Professor of
  Nursing Research
Wayne State University
Detroit, Michigan

Joan H. Baldwin, DNSc, RN
Associate Professor
Brigham Young University
Provo, Utah

**Elizabeth Ann Manhart Barrett,
  PhD, RN, FAAN**
Professor Emeriti
Hunter-Bellevue School of Nursing
Hunter College of the City
  University of New York
New York, New York

Kim Cameron, PhD, RN
Instructor
School of Nursing
University of Texas–Houston,
  Health Sciences Center
Houston, Texas

Kimberly F. Carter, PhD, RN
Associate Professor
Radford University
School of Nursing
Radford, Virginia

Marci Catanzaro, PhD, RN
was Research Associate Professor
  Emeritus
Biobehavioral Nursing & Health
  Science
University of Washington
Seattle, Washington

Julie Fleury, PhD, RN
Professor
College of Nursing
Arizona State University College
  of Nursing
Tempe, Arizona

Laurie Friedman Donze, PhD
Assistant Professor of Medicine
Johns Hopkins University School
  of Medicine
Baltimore, Maryland

Mattia J. Gilmartin, PhD, RN
Research Associate
Cambridge University of Health
The Judge Institute of
  Management Studies
Cambridge, United Kingdom

Judith Haber, PhD, RN, CS
Professor
New York University
Steinhardt School of Education,
  Division of Nursing
New York, New York

Rose M. Harvey, DNSc, RN
Adjunct Associate Professor of
  Nursing
Northeastern University
Boston, Massachusetts

Gail Hilbert-McAllister, DNSc, RN
Professor Emerita
The College of New Jersey
Union, New Jersey

Ann C. Hurley, DNSc, RN, FAAN
Executive Director
Center for Excellence in Nursing
    Practice
Brigham and Women's Hospital
Brookline, Massachusetts

Debra P. Hymovich, PhD, RN
Professor Emerita
College of Nursing and Health
    Professions
University of North Carolina at
    Charlotte
Charlotte, North Carolina

Anne Jalowiec, PhD, RN, FAAN
Professor Emerita
Loyola University of Chicago
Westmont, Illinois

Linda Corson Jones, PhD, RN
Deceased
Louisiana School of Nursing
Lousiana State University
New Orleans, Louisiana

Bessie Kirkwood, PhD
Professor
Department of Mathematical
    Sciences
Sweet Briar College
Sweet Briar, Virginia

Pamela A. Kulbok, DNSc, RN
Associate Professor
University of Virginia
School of Nursing
Charlottesville, Virginia

Cecile A. Lengacher, PhD, RN
Professor
University of South Florida
College of Nursing
Tampa, Florida

M. Cynthia Logsdon, DNS, ARNP
Associate Professor
University of Louisville
School of Nursing
Louisville, Kentucky

Ngozi O. Nkongho, PhD, RN
Chair, Department of Nursing
Lehman College—The City
    University of New York
Bronx, New York

Michael Perlow, DNS, RN
Associate Professor
Murray State University
Department of Nursing
Murray, Kentucky

Barbara Resnick, PhD, CRNP, FAAN
Assistant Professor
University of Maryland
School of Nursing
Baltimore, Maryland

Eric Sellers, MA
Graduate Research Assistant
University of South Florida
Tampa, Florida

Clarann Weinert, PhD, SC, RN, FAAN
Professor
Montana State University
College of Nursing
Bozeman, Montana

Gwen Wyatt, PhD, RN
Associate Professor
Michigan State University
College of Nursing
East Lansing, Michigan

Kate Yeager, MS, RN
Research Nurse
Rollins School of Public Health
Emory University
Atlanta, Georgia

PART I
Self-Efficacy and Self-Care

1

Self-Efficacy for Functional Activities Scale

Barbara Resnick

This chapter discusses the Self-Efficacy for Functional Activities scale, a measure of an individual's confidence in his or her ability to perform various functional activities, such as bathing and dressing.

PURPOSE

Self-efficacy is behavior-specific and dynamic in that it is focused on beliefs about personal abilities in a specific setting or with regard to a particular behavior, such as dieting or exercise. Because self-efficacy is highly context or situation dependent, measurement tools must be developed with respect to a specific task or activity. Self-efficacy expectations for functional activities are defined operationally by having the individual rate his or her perceived judgment or confidence in his or her ability to perform a specific activity of daily living at a given point in time. Measurement of self-efficacy expectations related to functional activities can be used to predict actual performance of activities of daily living and to identify those individuals with low self-efficacy expectations or motivation. Once these individuals are identified, appropriate interventions can be implemented to strengthen self-efficacy expectations related to functional activities and thereby improve functional performance.

CONCEPTUAL FRAMEWORK

The theory of self-efficacy is based on social cognitive theory, which attempts to predict and explain behavior using several key concepts, among which are outcome and self-efficacy expectations. Self-efficacy expectations are defined as an individual's judgment of his or her capabilities to organize and execute courses of action (Bandura, 1997). Judgments of self-efficacy also determine the degree of effort an individual will invest and the length of time a person will persist in a given activity. It is suggested that the stronger an individual's perceived self-efficacy, the more vigorous and persistent his or her efforts (Bandura, 1997; Bandura & Adams, 1977). In making a judgment of self-efficacy, Bandura (1997) identified four sources of efficacy information that influence the individual: (1) enactive attainment, (2) verbal persuasion, (3) vicarious experience, and (4) physiological or affective states such as pain or fatigue.

Operationalization of self-efficacy expectation is based on Bandura's (1977) early work with snake phobias. This approach included a paper-and-pencil measure that listed activities, from least to most difficult, in a specific behavioral domain. The respondents first indicated whether or not they could perform the activity (magnitude of self-efficacy), then evaluated the degree of confidence they had in performing the given activity (strength of self-efficacy). Respondents were given a 100-point scale, divided into 10-unit intervals ranging from 0 *(completely uncertain)* to 10, *(completely certain),* to identify the extent of confidence they had in performing the activity.

PROCEDURES FOR DEVELOPMENT

Items for the Self-Efficacy for Functional Activities (SEFA) scale were identified based on commonly recognized activities of daily living in older adults (Heinemann, Linacre, Wright, Hamilton, & Granger, 1994; Mahoney & Barthel, 1965). Specifically, these functional activities included eating, bathing, dressing, toileting, transferring, ambulation, and stair climbing. It was further recognized that these activities were performed (1) with the help of another person, (2) with adaptive equipment (i.e., cane, walker, reachers, long-handled sponges, or sock donners), or (3) independently. The SEFA scale initially included 27 items focusing on self-efficacy expectations related to performance of each activity at the three levels of ability.

Content validity of the SEFA was tested using two expert judges and an acceptable content validity index (CVI) of .80 (Waltz, Strickland, & Lenz, 1991). The two experts were a physician familiar with rehabilitation, self-efficacy, and principles of measurement and a nurse researcher familiar with self-efficacy measures. The nurse had also completed research using the theory of self-efficacy and was knowledgeable about measurement in nursing research. Both experts were given a blueprint, which included the behavioral objectives, content that guided the development of the tool, and a separate list of test items. The experts were asked to consider the objectives and content area of the measures and rate the relevancy of the items to the content by assigning each item a score using a 4-point rating scale: 1 = *not relevant,* 2 = *somewhat relevant,* 3 = *quite relevant,* and 4

= *very relevant.* Additionally, the raters were asked to include any items/ content they believed were needed to better assess the domain of interest. There was 100% agreement (CVI = 1.0) of the experts that the items were very relevant to self-efficacy expectations related to functional activities.

Initial pilot testing of the 27-item SEFA with a sample of 51 older adults who were participating in a rehabilitation program was done. Item analysis of the 27 items indicated that the 9 items related to performing the specific functional activity task with the help of another person were too easy (item difficulty score = 1.00) (Waltz et al., 1991), and the 5 items related to performing transfer and ambulation activities independently (i.e., with no assistive device) were too difficult (item difficulty score of 0). Participants believed that they were capable of performing all of the activities with the help of another person, and they needed to use an assistive device for ambulation and transfers. Therefore, the SEFA scale was shortened from 27 items to 9 items. The nine items focused on self-efficacy expectations related to performance of each activity of daily living either independently or with an assistive device. The revised 9-item measure combined 2 items for each functional activity from the 27-item measure and dropped the items related to performance with the help of another person (see Appendix).

DESCRIPTION

The SEFA scale is a 9-item measure that asks participants to rate their confidence in their ability to perform functional activities (with or without an assistive device). Specifically, these activities include bathing, dressing, transferring, toileting, ambulating, and climbing stairs. Generally, self-efficacy measures are ordered hierarchically from the easiest to the most difficult. There is, however, individual variation with regard to which functional task is the most difficult to perform. Therefore, random ordering of the items in the SEFA was done. Empirically, there was no difference in self-efficacy expectations when random ordering was done as opposed to placing items in order of increasing difficulty (Bandura, 1989).

Two formats can be used to measure self-efficacy expectations. The dual-judgment format involves having the individual first state whether or not he or she can execute the given activity (i.e., measuring magnitude of self-efficacy), and, if so, then rate the strength of his or her perceived efficacy. In the single-judgment format, the individual simply rates the strength of his or her perceived efficacy. The single-judgment format was used for this measure as it provides the same information and is generally easier to use (Bandura, 1995; Lee & Bobko, 1994).

ADMINISTRATION AND SCORING

The SEFA scale was administered using an interview format. Participants were instructed to listen to the statement, then use numbers from 0 to 10, with 0 being *no confidence* and 10 being *very confident*, to rate present beliefs in their ability to perform functional activities. The scale was scored by summing the numerical ratings for each activity and dividing by the number of activities. Self-efficacy was rated before any other scale was given to participants that might influence their self-efficacy expectations. In addition, only participants who could realistically perform the activity in question were invited to participate in the study. Otherwise it is a measure of wishful thinking, rather than a belief in one's ability to perform a behavior.

RELIABILITY AND VALIDITY EVIDENCE

Evidence of reliability and validity of the SEFA is described in Table 1.1.

CONCLUSION AND RECOMMENDATIONS

These studies provide some beginning evidence for the reliability and validity of the SEFA scale when used with older adults in a rehabilitation program and with those living in a long-term care facility. Reliability testing was based on internal consistency using alpha coefficients and test-retest reliability. Internal consistency of the measure indicated that there was consistency of responses across the items. The high alpha coefficients suggested that performance on any one item of the instrument was a good indicator of performance on any other item of the instrument. Test-retest reliability of the SEFA provided evidence for reliability when given in close temporal proximity.

To further assess the reliability of this measure, consideration should be given to use of an alternative estimate of reliability using a structured equations approach (Bollen, 1989). This approach is based on an alternative definition of reliability, which states that reliability of X (test score) is "the magnitude of the direct relations that all variables have on X" (Bollen, 1989, p. 54). Using a measurement model and structural equation modeling, a squared multiple correlation coefficient R^2 (Bollen, 1989) is calculated as the estimate of reliability. Specifically, R^2 provides a gauge of the systematic variance in the observed score that can be explained by each item in the measurement model (Bollen, 1989; Jagodzinski & Kuhnel, 1987; Reuterberg & Gustafsson, 1992). This approach overcomes issues identified in classical test theory such as the lack of recognition of

TABLE 1.1 Reliability and Validity Testing of the Self-efficacy for Functional Ability Scale (SEFA)

Study citation	Sample and characteristics	Reliability evidence	Validity evidence

Study 1: Pilot testing of the SEFA (Resnick, 1996.)	*Sample size:* 51
	 Sample characteristics:
	 Age: 77.7 ± 8.1
	 Gender:
	  Male 11 (22%)
	  Female 40 (78%)
	 Marital status
	  Married 20 (39%)
	  Widowed 30 (59%)
	  Never married 1 (2%)
	 Race:
	  Caucasian 44 (86%)
	  African American 7 (14%)
		Internal consistency:
		 Alpha of .81
		 Item ranges for item-to-total correlations: range .002 to .69
		 Interitem correlations: range .003 to .83
		 Test-retest: $r = .87$ (repeat testing done within 24 hours)
			Content validity:
			 Items generated from prior research and functional measures. CVI was 100, indicating 100% agreement of reviewers that the items were appropriate
			 Concurrent validity:
			 The Functional Inventory Measure (Heinneman et al., 1994) was used as the criterion; correlation of .49 on admission and .59 on discharge.
			 Predictive validity:
			 The Functional Inventory Measure (Heinneman et al., 1994) was used as the criterion, correlation of .30.
			 Construct validity:
			 It was hypothesized that SEFA would increase following rehabilitation.
			 Based on repeated measures, there was an increase in SEFA between admission and discharge ($F = 192$, $p < .05$).
			 Correlation of .30.

TABLE 1.1 (*continued*)

Study citation	Sample and characteristics	Reliability evidence	Validity evidence
Study 2: Resnick (1998a)	*Sample size:* 77 *Sample characteristics:* Age: 78.0 ± 7.2 Gender: Male 22 (29%) Female 55 (71%) Race: Caucasian 63 (82%) African American 14 (18%)	*Internal consistency:* Alpha of .84 to .88 (admission and discharge) Item ranges for item-to-total correlations: range .30 to .84 Interitem correlations: range .23 to .79	*Concurrent validity:* The Functional Inventory Measure (Heinneman et al., 1994) was used as the criterion. Correlation of .59 on admission and .69 on discharge. *Predictive validity:* The Functional Inventory Measure (Heinneman et al., 1994) was used as the criterion. Controlling for age and admission performance, the SEFA predicted discharge function (R^2 change = 3%, beta = .22, t = 2.0, p < .05).
Study 3: Resnick (1998b)	*Sample size:* 44 *Sample characteristics:* Age: 88.0 ± 6.4 Gender: Male 7 (16%) Female 37 (84%)	*Internal consistency:* Alpha of .92 Item ranges for item-to-total correlations: range .46 to .92. Interitem correlations: range .22 to .87.	*Concurrent validity:* The Functional Inventory Measure (Heinneman et al., 1994) was used as the criterion. Correlation of .88.

TABLE 1.1 (*continued*)

Study citation	Sample and characteristics	Reliability evidence	Validity evidence
Study 3: Resnick (1998b) (*continued*)	Race: Caucasian 44 (100%) Marital status Married 8 (12%) Widowed 50 (73%) Never married 11 (15%)		*Construct validity:* As hypothesized, individuals with depression (based on the Geriatric Depression Scale) had lower SEFA ($F = 4.2$, $p < .05$). As hypothesized, there was a positive correlation between motivation (based on the Apathy Evaluation Scale) and SEFA ($r = .49$, $p < .05$). $p < .05$) As hypothesized there was a negative correlation between fear of falling (based on a 0 to 4 scale) and SEFA ($r = -.30$, $p < .05$)

correlated errors of measurement and the indicators that are influenced by more than one latent variable.

These three studies provided evidence for the concurrent validity of the SEFA and as anticipated, less consistent support for the predictive validity of the measure. Self-efficacy expectations related to functional activities reflect the individual's motivation to perform these activities and theoretically will predict behavior, particularly behavior that is measured in close temporal proximity to self-efficacy expectations.

There also was support for the construct validity of the measure, suggesting that it can be used to identify those individuals with low self-efficacy expectations related to functional activities. These individuals can then be exposed to interventions to strengthen self-efficacy expectations, such as practicing the behavior, verbal persuasion, exposure to role models who successfully perform functional activities, and specific interventions to decrease the unpleasant physical sensations and affective states that are associated with the activity (Bandura, 1997; Resnick, 1996). Ultimately, this will help to improve performance of functional activities.

Construct validity is not determined by a single empirical test, and the findings from all three studies are important in the assessment of the construct validity of the SEFA scale. Study 3 provided additional evidence for the construct validity of the SEFA scale by supporting the hypothesized significant negative relationships between SEFA and fear of falling and depression, and the statistically significant positive relationship between the SEFA and the Apathy Evaluation Scale. More importantly, the results of Study 3 suggest that the SEFA scale is a reliable and valid measure for older adults in long-term care settings as well as those in rehabilitation programs. Continued research is needed to test the reliability and validity of this measure with other samples of older adults, such as those who are living in the community. Continued testing of the SEFA scale will further ensure that this measure is (1) consistent over time, and that the items have a direct relationship with the latent variable self-efficacy for functional activities; and (2) truly measures self-efficacy for functional activities.

REFERENCES

Bandura, A. (1977). Self-efficacy: Toward a unifying theory of behavioral change. *Psychological Review, 84,* 191–215.

Bandura, A. (1989). Regulation of cognitive processes through perceived self-efficacy. *Developmental Psychology, 25,* 725–729.

Bandura, A. (1995). *Self-efficacy in changing societies.* New York: Cambridge University Press.

Bandura, A. (1997). *Self-efficacy: The exercise of control.* New York: W. H. Freeman.

Bandura, A., & Adams, N. (1977). Analysis of self-efficacy theory of behavioral change. *Cognitive Therapy and Research, 1,* 287–304.

Bollen, K. (1989). *Structural equations with latent variables.* New York: Wiley.

Heinemann, A., Linacre, J., Wright, B., Hamilton, B., & Granger, C. (1994). Prediction of rehabilitation outcomes with disability measures. *Achieves of Physical Medicine and Rehabilitation, 75,* 133–143.

Jagodzinski, W., & Kuhnel, S. (1987). Estimation of reliability and stability in single-indicator multiple-wave models. *Sociological Methods and Research, 15,* 219–258.

Lee, C., & Bobko, P. (1994). Self-efficacy beliefs: comparison of five measures. *Journal of Applied Psychology, 79,* 364–369.

Mahoney, F., & Barthel, D. (1965). Functional evaluation: The Barthel Index. *Maryland State Medical Journal, 14*(2), 61–65.

Resnick, B. (1996). *Self-efficacy in geriatric rehabilitation.* Unpublished doctoral dissertation, University of Maryland, College Park, MD.

Resnick, B. (1998a). Efficacy beliefs in geriatric rehabilitation. *Journal of Gerontological Nursing, 24*(7), 34–44.

Resnick, B. (1998b). Functional performance of older adults in a long term care setting. *Clinical Nursing Research, 7,* 230–249.

Reuterberg, S., & Gustafsson, J. (1992). Confirmatory factor analysis and reliability: Testing measurement model assumptions. *Educational and Psychological Measurement, 52,* 795–811.

Waltz, C., Strickland, O., & Lenz, E. (1991). *Measurement in nursing research.* Philadelphia: F. A. Davis.

APPENDIX: SELF-EFFICACY FOR FUNCTIONAL ACTIVITIES SCALE

1. How confident are you that you can wash your upper body?

No Confidence   Total Confidence

0	1	2	3	4	5	6	7	8	9	10

2. How confident are you that you can wash your lower body?

0	1	2	3	4	5	6	7	8	9	10

3. How confident are you that you can dress your upper body?

0	1	2	3	4	5	6	7	8	9	10

4. How confident are you that you can dress your lower body?

0	1	2	3	4	5	6	7	8	9	10

5. How confident are you that you can get on and off the toilet and manage your clothes?

0	1	2	3	4	5	6	7	8	9	10

6. How confident are you that you can get in and out of bed and a chair?

0	1	2	3	4	5	6	7	8	9	10

7. How confident are you that you can walk (50ft)?

0	1	2	3	4	5	6	7	8	9	10

8. How confident are you that you can walk (120ft)?

0	1	2	3	4	5	6	7	8	9	10

9. How confident are you that you can climb up and down 4 stairs?

0	1	2	3	4	5	6	7	8	9	10

2

The Perlow Self-Esteem Scale

Michael Perlow

This chapter discusses the Perlow Self-Esteem Scale, a measure of self-esteem based on Coopersmith's theory of self-esteem.

PURPOSE

Self-esteem is a construct that has generated a good deal of interest in the past three decades. While discussion and utilization of self-esteem has been rather widespread, progress in clarifying and assessing the construct has lagged. O'Brien (1980) considered a distinct theoretical link to be a necessary component of self-esteem. In addition O'Brien believed that methodologic rigor in validation is a necessary component of any self-esteem measure. Wylie (1974, 1979) also called for methodologic rigor and distinct theoretical links in determining the validity of any self-esteem measure.

To follow the recommendations of O'Brien (1980) and Wylie (1974, 1979), Perlow (1987, 1990, 1992) developed and examined the Perlow Self-Esteem Scale (PSES) based on the potentially enlightening theory of self-esteem from Stanley Coopersmith (1981). Although a variety of self-esteem instruments already exist, the development of the PSES was seen as significant because the PSES was designed to have a distinct theoretical link, an aspect missing in many of the previous attempts to measure this construct (Wylie, 1974, 1979). Additionally, the development of a brief, easy-to-use instrument feasible for clinical settings was desirable.

THEORETICAL FRAMEWORK

Coopersmith's (1981) theory describing self-esteem has four constructs: values, aspirations, and defenses. Four additional constructs—power, significance, virtue, and competence—are subsumed under success. Each of the concepts, as well as self-esteem, is described in the following paragraphs.

Success

Coopersmith's (1981) theory selected success from the writings of William James (1890/1981) as one aspect of self-esteem. Success to both James and Coopersmith is one's perception of achievement and as such is internally defined. Although this achievement tends to be similar in individuals of a similar culture, the perception of success is entirely personal and not dependent on any external criteria. Coopersmith further described success with four dimensions as follows: power, significance, virtue, and competence. Power is one's ability to control behavior, both one's own and that of others. Significance is the acceptance and popularity given an individual by others. Virtue is adherence to a prescribed set of ethics, and competence is the individual's level of achievement. That is to say, a successful person is one who has considerable competence and power, has high standards, and is well accepted by others.

Values

As with success, this construct was taken from the work of James (1890). Values are those measures of importance that an individual attaches to a situation. These values arise from social norms and as with success are consistent within similar cultures. The social context of these values becomes so firmly entrenched that any personal values that deviate from the social have minimal effect (Coopersmith, 1981).

Aspirations

This third construct was again from the work of James (1890/1981). Aspirations are the goals individuals establish for themselves. These goals arise from two sources: personal or public. Personal goals vary with each individual, whereas public goals are consistent throughout a culture (Coopersmith, 1981).

Defenses

The final construct was included by Coopersmith (1981) from the work of H. S. Sullivan (1953). Defense was defined differently than the popular use of defenses arising from psychoanalytic theory's "defense mechanisms." In this context, defense refers to the ability to resist devaluation to one's self-esteem.

Self-Esteem

Self-esteem is the perception of success weighted against values, measured against aspirations, and filtered through defenses (Coopersmith, 1981).

Coopersmith (1981) offered three stated relationships among the four concepts of success, values, aspirations, and defenses. The relationship statements are as follows:

1. As success increases, self-esteem increases.
2. As self-esteem increases, aspirations increase.
3. As self-esteem increases, defenses increase.

A fourth relationship statement may be inferred from the conceptual definition of success and the relationship between success and self-esteem. The inferred relationship is as follows:

4. As power, significance, virtue, and competence increase, self-esteem increases.

PROCEDURES FOR DEVELOPMENT

In order to do justice to and adequately test Coopersmith's (1981) theory, three items were developed from each of the four constructs—power, significance, virtue, and competence—that Coopersmith employed to describe success. In addition, three items were developed for each of the remaining constructs—values, aspirations, and defenses—by which Coopersmith defined self-esteem. The initial PSES, therefore, consisted of 21 items, 3 drawn from each of Coopersmith's constructs.

Each of the items was a simple statement the respondents were to select as being either like or unlike themselves. The items were created to sample the domain of self-esteem because they were written following Coopersmith's (1981) constructs. Once developed, the items were submitted to a panel of individuals familiar with Coopersmith's theory. This panel concurred that the items reflected the essence of the constructs, thereby providing evidence for content validity of the PSES.

An alpha extraction with varimax rotation factor analysis was conducted on the 21 items of the PSES, with a minimum loading of 0.40 defining a factor. Two factors emerged, one consisting of 17 items reflecting internal self and one consisting of 4 items that reflected external self. Consistent with Coopersmith's (1981) perspective, the 17 items reflecting the internal self were chosen for the PSES, and the 4 items reflecting external self were discarded (Perlow, 1987).

TABLE 2.1 Perlow Self-Esteem Scale

Those indicated "X" are reverse-scored.	5	4	3	2	1
I have high standards for my behavior.					
My life is out of control.	X				
I have realistic values.					
I have big plans.					
My values are not well defined.	X				
I have control of my life.					
People like me for what I am.					
I have stable values.					
I am virtuous.					
My standards are less than others' standards.	X				
People pay attention to me.					
I can control my anxiety.					
People do not always understand the real me.	X				
I am able to achieve what I desire.					
I can't get what I want.	X				
My aims are high.					
I am able to influence others.					

5–Like me   2–Somewhat unlike me
4–Somewhat like me   1–Unlike me
3–Neither like me or unlike me

DESCRIPTION, ADMINISTRATION, AND SCORING

The instrument consists of 17 printed statements. The respondents are instructed to indicate how each of the 17 statements is either like or unlike them. They are requested to choose their responses on the basis of their feelings and are further informed that there are no right or wrong answers.

The responses are recorded on a 5-point Likert-type scale. The divisions of the Likert-type scale are from 5 (*like me*) to 1 (*unlike me*). Statements representing positive self-esteem are scored 5 points (*like me*) to 1 point (*unlike me*). Statements representing negative self-esteem are reverse-scored. The reverse-scored items are 2, 5, 10, 13, and 15. The item values are then summed to provide a total score for each respondent. The higher the score, the higher the respondent's self-esteem, with a potential score range from 85 to 17. A copy of the PSES is provided in Table 2.1.

RELIABILITY AND VALIDITY

Three different studies that examined the reliability and validity of the PSES are provided in this section. The studies are sequenced according to the time of their completion rather than the date of their publication.

Study 1

To test the discrimination of the PSES, two different groups of individuals assumed to have different levels of self-esteem were solicited to participate in the study (Perlow, 1992). One group consisted of individuals belonging to and participating in philanthropic groups and were therefore assumed to have high self-esteem. The mean age of this group was 37.37 years, and the number of years in school was 16.81 years. The other group consisted of individuals who were participants in self-help groups, were dissatisfied with some aspect of their self, and were assumed to have low self-esteem. The mean age of this group was 45.65 years, and the mean years in school was 14 years.

Respondents completed three measures of self-esteem: the PSES, Coopersmith's Adult Form Self-Esteem Inventory (SEI), and a semantic differential (SD) scale designed to measure self-esteem.

Reliability

The PSES had a Cronbach's alpha of .86. The Pearson product–moment correlation coefficient for 57 individuals who completed a 30-day retest of the PSES was $r = .84$. The PSES therefore demonstrated both internal consistency and stability.

Validity

Two different approaches were used to assess validity. Concurrent validity was assessed by obtaining the Pearson product–moment correlation coefficients between the PSES and the SEI and SD, two instruments with previous evidence of validity (Coopersmith, 1981; Perlow, 1987). The Pearson product–moment coefficient between the PSES and the SEI was $r = .78$, and the Pearson coefficient between the PSES and the SD was $r = .68$, with both values being statistically significant. The PSES therefore demonstrated concurrent validity.

To test that the PSES would discriminate between the two groups, a one-way analysis of variance comparing PSES scores from the two groups was obtained. The PSES did discriminate between the two groups $F(1,110) = 10.08$, $p < .002$, thus supporting construct validity of the PSES. Both the

SEI and SD also discriminated between the groups, providing evidence supporting the initial assumption of group differences in self-esteem.

Study 2

Perlow (1990) further assessed reliability and validity of the PSES with 98 respondents who completed the PSES and Zung's (1971) Self Report Anxiety Scale (SAS). The mean age of this sample was 27.93 years ($SD =$ 10.10), and the mean education was 14.85 years ($SD = 1.77$).

Reliability

The PSES had a Cronbach's alpha of .81. A Pearson product–moment correlation coefficient for a 30-day test-retest for 66 of the original subjects was $r = .51$. The PSES again demonstrated internal consistency and stability.

Validity

Because Sullivan (1953) and later Coopersmith (1981) believed there was an inverse relationship between self-esteem and anxiety, two hypotheses were tested as follows: (1) An inverse relationship exists between PSES and SAS scores, and (2) two groups defined by the top and bottom of SAS scores will have different levels of self-esteem. To test the first hypothesis, a Pearson product–moment correlation coefficient was obtained between PSES and SAS scores. The coefficient was significant at $r = -.38$, thereby supporting construct validity of the PSES.

   To test the second hypothesis, the respondents were divided into two groups according to their SAS scores. The mean SAS score was 34.62. Those individuals selected for the high-anxiety group had scores greater than 35, whereas those individuals selected for the low-anxiety group had scores less than 34. To test for differences, a one-way analysis of variance was obtained on PSES scores between the two groups $F(1,85) = 9.31$, $p <$ .003. Because of the significant group differences, the second hypothesis, and therefore PSES construct validity, was supported.

Study 3

Bryant (1988) employed the PSES to estimate validity for a newly developed tool designed to measure acceptance of self. Twenty-three individuals completed the prepilot study, and 18 completed the pilot study. During both of the data collection times, the respondents completed the Acceptance of Self scale and the PSES to test for the hypothesized positive relationship between self-esteem and self-acceptance. The prepilot study correlation coefficients involving the PSES were $r = .21$ for form 1 and $r = .45$ for form 2. Pilot study correlation coefficients involving the PSES were $r = .60$ for form 1 and $r = .59$ for form 2. The Acceptance of Self tool functioned as hypothesized and supported concurrent validity of the PSES.

CONCLUSIONS AND RECOMMENDATIONS

The PSES is an internally consistent measure of self-esteem. Stability of the PSES was demonstrated in the initial study but was not strongly supported in the subsequent study. Content validity of the PSES was claimed by means of the tool construction (Perlow, 1987), and concurrent validity was supported by comparisons of the PSES with the SEI and SD (Perlow, 1992). Construct validity was supported by factor analysis of the items (Perlow, 1987) and hypothesis testing (Perlow, 1990, 1992).

Although a new instrument, the PSES has maintained its claim to internal consistency and stability. In addition, the PSES has demonstrated content, concurrent, and construct validity. The implications of a reliable and valid measure of self-esteem for nursing are readily evident. Self-esteem is directly related to the psychological well-being of the individual. Behaviors arising from interpersonal interactions are affected by self-esteem, and the effect of psychological constructs on the physical self is just beginning to be examined.

The value of a tool like the PSES, with few items, is especially significant. Because of its brevity and simplicity, use of the PSES in clinical settings would likely invoke less resistance from health care providers and greater acceptance from recipients of health care. The encouraging results and the obvious advantages of the PSES warrant further testing.

Additional testing of the PSES is warranted. Particularly the stability of the tool needs to be resolved. An extensive factor analysis should be undertaken to examine the underlying structure of the PSES. Additional concurrent comparisons as well as hypothesis testing should be undertaken to provide additional information about the function of the PSES.

REFERENCES

Bryant, S. (1988, March). *Development of an instrument to measure acceptance of self.* Paper presented at the Measurement of Clinical and Educational Nursing Outcomes Conference, San Diego, CA.

Coopersmith, S. (1981). *The antecedents of self-esteem.* Palo Alto, CA: Consulting Psychologist Press.

James, W. (1890/1981). *The principles of psychology* (Vol.1). New York: Holt. (Original work published 1890)

O'Brien, E. J. (1980). The self-report inventory: Development and validation of a multi-dimensional measure of the self-concept and sources of self-esteem. *Dissertation Abstracts International, 41,* 3191B–3192B.

Perlow, M. (1987). Coopersmith's adult form self-esteem inventory: A construct validation study. *Dissertation Abstracts International, 49,* 3679B.

Perlow, M. (1990). The Perlow self-esteem scale. In C. Waltz & O. Strickland (Eds.), *Measurement of nursing outcomes: Measuring client self-care and coping skills* (pp. 135–146). New York: Springer.

Perlow, M. (1992). Validity and reliability of the PSES. *Western Journal of Nursing Research, 14,* 201–210.

Sullivan, H. S. (1953). *The interpersonal theory of psychiatry.* New York: Norton.

Wylie, R. (1974). *The self-concept* (Vol. 1 rev.ed.). Lincoln: University of Nebraska Press.

Wylie, R. (1979). *The self-concept* (Vol. 2). Lincoln: University of Nebraska Press.

Zung, W. (1971). A rating instrument for anxiety disorders. *Psychosomatics, 12,* 371–379.

3

A Measure of Power as Knowing Participation in Change

Elizabeth Ann Manhart Barrett

This chapter discusses the Power as Knowing Participation in Change Tool, a measure of one's perceived power.

PURPOSE

The Power as Knowing Participation in Change Tool (PKPCT) was developed to measure power defined as the capacity to participate knowingly in the nature of change as manifest by awareness (A), choices (C), freedom to act intentionally (F), and involvement in creating change (I) (Barrett, 1983, 1986, 1990a). Rogers' (1970, 1992) science of unitary human beings postulates that humans can knowingly participate in change. From this axiom, Barrett derived a new theory of power and developed an instrument to measure the theoretical power construct. The tool is designed for use with men and women 18 and older in various settings.

A minimum of a high school education is required due to the literacy level of the adjectives.

CONCEPTUAL BASIS OF THE POWER AS KNOWING PARTICIPATION IN CHANGE TOOL

Guided by Rogers' (1970, 1992) science, the power theory and the PK-PCT are consistent with the postulates of energy fields, openness, pattern, and pandimensionality, as well as the principles of helicy, resonancy, and integrality. This acausal theory is differentiated from other power theories that postulate power to be the ability to cause or prevent change (May, 1972).

Hence, this theory is about power as freedom, not power as control. It is proposed that individuals or groups can knowingly participate in creating their reality; yet concurrently, other individuals or groups as well as all else in the environment are also participating, knowingly or unknowingly. Thus, control is an illusion; there is only the capacity to participate in change in a knowing and powerful manner.

Power as knowing participation is being aware of what one is choosing to do, feeling free to do it, and doing it intentionally. Awareness and freedom to act intentionally guide choices and involvement in creating changes. It is the continuously shifting dynamic mix of A, C, F, and I that constitutes power. Power is freedom to make aware choices regarding involvement in life situations, including health-promoting changes. Depending on the nature of that awareness and the strength of the choices one makes, and how free one feels to act on intentions, the range of situations in which one is involved in creating changes and the manner in which one knowingly participates vary (Barrett, 1983, 1986, 1989, 1990b). Feeling free to act as one wishes is critical to power, because it impacts on the potency as well as the kinds of choices one makes, including choosing the particular changes one is involved in creating.

The theoretical definitions of the subscales of the PKPCT are based on the central concepts, or the four power dimensions in the conceptual framework. *Awareness* is the focusing of attention on what one perceives to exist. *Choices* are selections from possibilities for participating in experiences. *Freedom to act intentionally* is the experience of one's capacity to do or bring about what one has in mind. *Involvement in creating change* is innovative engagement in the unpredictable human–environment mutual process to actualize some potentials rather than others.

Power is neither good nor evil in and of itself, although we as individuals or groups can label the form in which power manifests as constructive or destructive. The intensity, frequency, and form in which power manifests vary. The changes are innovative, creative, and unpredictable (Barrett, 1986, 1989).

The inseparable association of the four power dimensions is the individual or group power profile. Changes in the power profile are nonlinear and indicate (1) the nature of the awareness of experiences, (2) the type of choices made, (3) the degree to which freedom to act intentionally is operating, and (4) the manner of involvement in creating specific changes. The PKPCT provides an estimate of the power profile (Barrett, 1983, 1990b).

PROCEDURES FOR DEVELOPMENT

Procedures for development consisted of three phases: judges' studies, a pilot study, and a validation study (Barrett, 1990a). Each phase will be discussed briefly.

Judges' Studies

Nursing faculty who were considered knowledgeable concerning Rogers' science of unitary human beings served as judges in two ($n = 5$, $n = 4$) studies. Based on a given description of the beginning power theory, judges used a checklist to indicate words or phrases that were theoretically consistent. Next, using a 7-point semantic differential, judges rated 43 bipolar adjective pairs according to the theory and Rogers' science. In the second study, faculty used Likert scaling technique to rate four concepts that characterized the dimensions of power (A, C, F, I) and three contexts (self, family, occupation). Next, a semantic differential approach was used to rate 38 bipolar adjective pairs. In summary, the 7-point semantic differential technique was used to construct a power measure comprised of 4 concepts, 3 contexts, and 24 scales.

Pilot Study

A national volunteer sample that was diverse in terms of age, gender, marital status, city size, geographical residence, and occupation with a minimum of a high school education, was secured. Responses for each subject (n =267; response rate = 53%) on the concept–context scale combinations (4 concepts x 3 contexts x 24 scales = 288 variables) were placed in a single matrix and factor analyzed using principal components with varimax rotation (Maguire, 1973). Three factors with an eigenvalue greater than 1.0 emerged and accounted for 51% of the variance. Further factor analyses and congruence coefficients (.72 to .98 for the concepts; .86 to .98 for the contexts) indicated that neither concepts nor contexts differentiated scale responses, thus suggesting that power is a single dimension. Next, factor score means ($-.31$ to .17) were examined to select the most distinctively discriminating aspects of power. The revised instrument consisted of four concept–context combinations.

Validation Study

Responses from a similar national sample of participants from all states ($n = 625$; response rate 61%) were arranged in a single data matrix, and one factor with an eigenvalue greater than 1.0 emerged during factor analysis, which accounted for 43% of the variance. Factor score means revealed the same rank order as had occurred in the pilot study ($-.25$ to .22). Means for the scales ranged from 5.06 to 6.07 and suggested the tool had an inherent bias toward the high-frequency descriptors and possibly social desirability response set.

Congruence coefficients of .99 again provided evidence that power generalized across contexts. Therefore, a second form of the instrument was proposed; the four concepts are rated without the modifying contexts. This tool, the PKPCT, Version II has subsequently been used by the majority of researchers investigating power as knowing participation in change.

DESCRIPTION

The PKPCT is a 7-point semantic differential type of instrument. Semantic differential technique was used to measure the meaning of the operational indicators of power, manifested by awareness (A), choices (C), freedom to act intentionally (F), and involvement in creating change (I). These concepts comprise 4 subscales rated against 12 bipolar adjective scales and 1 retest reliability item. Osgood's semantic differential type of measurement has been shown to be reliable and valid, lends itself to statistical techniques for validation purposes, is uncomplicated, and requires a short amount of time to complete (Osgood, Suci, & Tannenbaum, 1957).

Version I uses 12 bipolar adjective pairs and 1 repeat adjective pair as a retest reliability or acquiescence scale to rate 4 concept–context combinations: awareness in relation to occupation, choices in relation to myself, freedom to act intentionally in relations with family, and involvement in creating changes in relations with family. The same bipolar adjectives are randomly ordered for each concept–context. Version II is identical except that concepts are rated without the concept–context combinations as awareness, choices, freedom to act intentionally, and involvement in creating change. The word *power* does not appear on the instrument as an attempt to prevent bias.

ADMINISTRATION AND SCORING

Recently, the instruments were reprinted with revised instructions, based on a research study (Barrett, Farren, Kim, Larkin, & Mahoney, 2001). For each concept–context (Version I) or concept (Version II), participants are instructed to make a separate rating with each bipolar adjective pair and to check the space that best reflects the meaning for them. Administration does not require a face-to-face data collection procedure. However, this approach is preferred because it allows for standardizing test conditions.

Although factor scores allow for greater measurement precision, scale scores can be summed. The range is 12 to 84 for each power concept–context or concept and 48 to 336 for the total power score. Lower scores indicate lower power; higher scores indicate higher power. Although reversed randomly throughout the instrument, the adjectives indicating higher power are as follows: profound, seeking, valuable, intentional, assertive, leading, orderly, expanding, pleasant, informed, free, important. Versions I and II of the PKPCT and the scoring guide for Version 2 appear in the Appendix. Version I is scored in a manner similar to Version II. Use of the tool requires permission from the author.*

RELIABILITY AND VALIDITY EVIDENCE

Reliability

Reliability was initially reported as the variance of factor scores and ranged from .55 to .99 in the pilot study and from .63 to .99 in the validation study. Barrett and other researchers have since used Cronbach's alpha procedure to assess internal consistency, and reliabilities most often have been above .85 (Barrett, Caroselli, Sullivan Smith, & Woods Smith, 1997). A review of 39 studies of power is reported in the literature and includes detailed descriptions of the research, including psychometric properties of the PKPCT (Caroselli & Barrett, 1998).

The last bipolar adjective pair on each power dimension is used to calculate item retest reliability (with a reported range from .38 to .91), or it can be used as an acquiescor scale (with 91% to 99% of responses representing no more than 1 point difference, with the maximum of 6 possible point differences) (Barrett & Caroselli, 1998). Test–retest reliability (n = 25) of the PKPCT was assessed with a 3-week interval; correlations ranged from .71 to .82 for Version 1 and .61 to .78 for Version 2 (Barrett, 1996).

Validity

The judges' studies provided a priori content validity for the PKPCT. In the validation study, construct validity was assessed using factor analysis with loadings ranging from .56 to .70 (Barrett, 1983, 1986). Nunnally (1978) maintains that factor loadings greater than .40 suggest construct validity. Factor analysis in Trangenstein's (1988) study provided further evidence of construct validity (Barrett & Caroselli, 1998).

In two studies, the PKPCT was used to estimate concurrent validity with instruments developed by those authors. Leddy (1995) reported a correlation of .65 between the Well-Being Index and the PKPCT, Version

---

*Contact the author at the following address for use of the tool: Elizabeth Ann Manhart Barrett, RN, PhD, FAAN, 415 East 85th Street, 9E, New York, New York 10028.

II and .69 between the Health Synchrony Scale and the PKPCT, Version II. Marsh (1989), using the Marsh Revelation Scale, found correlations with the PKPCT, Version I ranged from .19 to .43.

Hypothesis-testing studies that were analyzed by Caroselli and Barrett (1998) have provided evidence for construct validity in samples of healthy adults or clients/patients by demonstrating positive, statistically significant relationships between power (or a power subscale) and human field motion, life satisfaction, purpose in life, well-being, self-transcendence, spirituality, perspective taking, imagination, perceived health, and socioeconomic status and inverse relationships with personal distress, chronic pain, environmental factors, anxiety, previous crisis, injury severity, and hopelessness. Nurse-focused studies demonstrated significant relationships between power (or a power subscale) and leadership effectiveness, job diversity, feminism, transformational leadership, imagination, and empathy and inverse relationships with transactional leadership and creativity (Caroselli & Barrett, 1998, p. 14).

Further evidence of validity is suggested by the ability of the PKPCT to detect differences between experimental and control groups or between comparison groups, although further support is needed to more accurately assess this sensitivity. Also, keep in mind that as a consideration of construct validity, discrimination between groups concerns both theory and measurement (Thorndike & Hagan, 1977). Therefore, the lack of differences between groups may be due to faulty theorizing.

Higher power was demonstrated in persons who reduced smoking versus persons who did not reduce smoking ($p = .05$) (Wynd, 1992), in reminiscence storytelling participants versus control group participants ($p = .05$) (Bramlett & Gueldner, 1993), in diabetics receiving education versus diabetics not receiving education ($p = .05$ (Roznowski, 1995), in Swedes and Finns versus Japanese and Koreans ($p = .05$) (Winstead-Fry et al., 1996), and in asthmatics who used guided imagery versus asthmatics who did not practice guided imagery ($p = .04$) (Epstein et al., 2001). Conversely, no significant difference between groups was detected in a different study of reminiscence storytelling participants versus control group participants (Bramlett, 1990), or in dyspneic patients receiving education versus a control group (Krause, 1991), or in postmenopausal women with coronary artery disease versus postmenopausal women without coronary artery disease (Gloss & Crowe, 1993), or in polio survivors versus persons with no comparable disease (Smith, 1995).

The PKPCT, Version 2 has been translated into Swedish, Finnish, Korean, and Japanese using the blind back-translation methodology (Winstead-Fry et al., 1996). The PKPCT was administered to 50 men and 50 women in each of these countries ($n = 400$). Means similar to those found in various populations in the United States supported the hypothesis that power as knowing participation in change is a universal phenomenon.

CONCLUSIONS AND RECOMMENDATIONS

The following conclusions are made regarding the psychometric evidence for the Power as Knowing Participation in Change Tool.

1. Congruence coefficients and factor structures suggested that power generalized across indices of the human (self) and environmental (family, occupation) fields. This supported the construct validity of the PKPCT as well as Rogers' (1970, 1992) proposition that the two fields, though different by definition, are integral with one another (Barrett, 1990a).
2. Consistent with the theory, age, gender, and education have not been important predictors of power (Caroselli & Barrett, 1998). These findings also support the construct validity of the PKPCT.
3. There is growing support for the reliability and validity of the PKPCT, Version I and the PKPCT, Version II (Caroselli & Barrett, 1998).
4. The predominant use of nonrandomly selected convenience samples limits the ability to generalize findings to other groups (Barrett & Caroselli, 1998).
5. In a review of 39 studies, the number of studies where hypotheses related to power were fully supported was more than double the number where hypotheses were partially supported or not supported (Caroselli & Barrett, 1998).

Based on results related to the PKPCT, the following recommendations are offered.

1. Meta-analysis of the quantitative power studies need to be conducted (Caroselli & Barrett, 1998).
2. Determination of norms for the PKPCT should be done to ascertain what scores represent lower, moderate, and higher power (Barrett & Caroselli, 1998).
3. Comparative studies using the known groups hypothesis testing technique are needed to further validate the PKPCT (Barrett & Caroselli, 1998).
4. Studies need to be designed to detect differences between groups using random assignment with matching on key variables and random sampling when possible (Barrett & Caroselli, 1998).
5. Cross-cultural research using the PKPCT needs to continue to test the proposition that power is a universal phenomenon (Caroselli & Barrett, 1998).
6. Research needs to continue that examines the relationship between power and age, gender, education, occupation, race, ethnicity, and socioeconomic status in a more critical manner.

In conclusion, there has been sufficient evidence gathered regarding the psychometric properties of the PKPCT that indicates it is a reliable and valid measure of power. It can be used with reasonable confidence as a measure of power in research and practice as well as in a variety of populations. However, further psychometric evaluation is warranted.

REFERENCES

Barrett, E. A. M. (1983). *An empirical investigation of Martha E. Rogers' principle of helicy: The relationship of human field motion and power.* Unpublished doctoral dissertation, New York University, New York.

Barrett, E. A. M. (1986). The principle of helicy: The relationship of human field motion and power. In V. M. Malinski (Ed.), *Explorations on Martha Rogers' science of unitary human beings* (pp. 173–188). Norwalk, CT: Appleton-Century-Crofts.

Barrett, E. A. M. (1989). A nursing theory of power for nursing practice: Derivation from Rogers' paradigm. In J. Riehl (Ed.), *Conceptual models for nursing practice* (3rd ed.), (pp. 207–217). Norwalk, CT: Appleton & Lange.

Barrett, E. A. M. (1990a). An instrument to measure power as knowing participation in change. In O. Strickland & C. Waltz (Eds.), *The measurement of nursing outcomes: Measuring client self-care and coping skills* (Vol. 4), (pp. 159–180). New York: Springer.

Barrett, E. A. M. (1990b). Health patterning with clients in a private practice environment. In E. A. M. Barrett (Ed.), *Visions of Rogers' science-based nursing* (pp. 105–115). New York: National League for Nursing.

Barrett, E. A. M. (1996). *The relationship of human field motion and power: A replication and extension.* Unpublished manuscript.

Barrett, E. A. M., & Caroselli, C. (1998). Methodological ponderings related to the power as knowing participation in change tool. *Nursing Science Quarterly, 11,* 17–22.

Barrett, E. A. M., Caroselli, C., Sullivan Smith, A., & Woods Smith, D. (1997). Power as knowing participation in change: Theoretical, practice, and methodological issues, insights, and ideas. In M. Madrid (Ed.), *Patterns of Rogerian knowing* (pp. 31–46). New York: National League for Nursing.

Barrett, E. A. M., Farren, A., Kim, T., Larkin, D., & Mahoney, J. (2001). A study of the PKPCT instructions. *Visions: The Journal of Rogerian Nursing Science, 9,* 61–65.

Bramlett, M. H. (1991). Power, creativity and reminiscence in the elderly. *Dissertation Abstracts International, 51*(07), 3317B, (UMN No. 9027677)

Bramlett, M. H., & Gueldener, S. H. (1993). Reminiscence: A viable option to enhance power in elders. *Clinical Nurse Specialist, 7*(2), 68–74.

Caroselli, C., & Barrett, E. A. M. (1998). A review of the power as knowing participation in change literature. *Nursing Science Quarterly, 11,* 9–16.

Epstein, G., Halper, J., Barrett, E. A. M., Birdsall, C., McGee, M., Baron, K. P., & Lowenstein, S. (2001). *A study of mind-body changes in adults with asthma who practice mental imagery.* Unpublished manuscript.

Gloss, E. F., & Crowe, R. L. (1993, June). Coronary artery disease: Postmenopausal women, power, and anxiety. *Proceedings of the Sigma Theta Tau International Research Congress, Advances in International Nursing.*

Krause, D. A. B. (1991). *The impact of an individually tailored nursing intervention on human field patterning of patients experiencing dyspnea.* Unpublished doctoral dissertation, University of Miami, Miami, Florida.

Leddy, S. K. (1995). Measuring mutual process: Development and psychometric testing of the person-environment participation scale. *Visions: The Journal of Rogerian Nursing Science, 3*(1), 20–31.

Maguire, T. O. (1973). Semantic differential methodology for the structuring of attitudes. *American Education Research Journal, 10,* 295–306.

Marsh, G. M. (1989). *The development and testing of instruments to measure concepts in the revelation readiness model of lifestyle change.* Unpublished doctoral dissertation, University of Arizona, Tucson.

May, R. (1972). *Power and innocence.* New York: Dell.

Nunnally, J. C. (1978). *Psychometric theory* (2nd ed.). New York: McGraw-Hill.

Osgood, C. E, Suci, C. J., & Tannenbaum, P. H. (1957). *The measurement of meaning.* Chicago: University of Illinois Press.

Rogers, M. E. (1970). *An introduction to the theoretical basis of nursing.* Philadelphia: F. A. Davis.

Rogers, M. E. (1992). Nursing science and the space age. *Nursing Science Quarterly, 5,* 27–34.

Roznowski, H. (1995). *Diabetes education: Knowledge, power, and change.* Unpublished master's thesis, Northern Michigan University, Marquette.

Smith, D. W., (1995). Power and spirituality in polio survivors. *Nursing Science Quarterly, 8,* 133–139.

Thorndike, R. L., & Hagan, E. P. (1977). *Measurement and evaluation in psychology and education* (4th ed.). New York: Wiley.

Trangenstein, P. A. (1988). *The relationships of power and diversity to job satisfaction and job involvement: An empirical investigation of Rogers' principle of integrality.* Unpublished doctoral dissertation, New York University, New York.

Winstead-Fry, P., Paletta, J. L., Barrett, E. A. M., Krause, K., Lee, W. H., Nojima, Y., & Olsson, H. (1996). Transcultural exploration of measurement scales for the study of Rogers' conceptual model. *International Society of University Nurses Newsletter, 10*(2), 2.

Wynd, C. A. (1992). Personal power imagery and relaxation techniques used in smoking cessation programs. *American Journal of Health Promotion, 6,* 184–189, 196.

APPENDIX: BARRET'S PKPCT

INTRODUCTION TO BARRETT'S PKPCT

The PKPCT is designed to help you describe the meaning of day-to-day change in your life. Four indicators of experiencing change are:

> AWARENESS
> CHOICES
> FREEDOM TO ACT INTENTIONALLY
> INVOLVEMENT IN CREATING CHANGE

These indicators can also be described in relation to self, family, and occupation.
It takes about 10 minutes to complete the PKPCT.

INSTRUCTIONS FOR COMPLETING BARRETT'S PKPCT

For each indicator, there are 13 lines. There are words at both ends of each line. The meaning of the words are opposite to each other. There are 7 spaces between each pair of words which provide a range of possible responses. Place an "X" in the space along the line that best describes the meaning of the indicator (AWARENESS, CHOICES, FREEDOM TO ACT INTENTIONALLY, or INVOLVEMENT IN CREATING CHANGE) for you at this time.

For example:
Under the indicator CHOICES, if your CHOICES are quite closely described as "informed," your answer might look like this:

> informed ___|_X_|___|___|___|___|___| uninformed

If your CHOICES are quite closely described as "uninformed," your answer might look like this:

> informed ___|___|___|___|___|_X_|___ uninformed

If your CHOICES are equally "informed" and "uninformed," place an "X" in the middle space on the line. Your answer might look like this:

> informed ___|___|___|_X_|___|___|___ uninformed

REMEMBER:
- There are no right or wrong answers.
- Record your first impression for **each pair of words**.
- You can place an "X" in any space along the line that best describes the meaning the indicator has for you at this time.
- Mark only one "X" for each pair of words.
- Mark an "X" for every pair of words.

PLEASE BEGIN TO MARK YOUR X'S ON BARRETT'S PKPCT

BARRETT PKPCT, Version I

In relation to my OCCUPATION (work and/or school):
MY AWARENESS IS

profound	___	___	___	___	___	___	___	superficial
avoiding	___	___	___	___	___	___	___	seeking
valuable	___	___	___	___	___	___	___	worthless
unintentional	___	___	___	___	___	___	___	intentional
timid	___	___	___	___	___	___	___	assertive
leading	___	___	___	___	___	___	___	following
chaotic	___	___	___	___	___	___	___	orderly
expanding	___	___	___	___	___	___	___	shrinking
pleasant	___	___	___	___	___	___	___	unpleasant
uninformed	___	___	___	___	___	___	___	informed
free	___	___	___	___	___	___	___	constrained
unimportant	___	___	___	___	___	___	___	important
unpleasant	___	___	___	___	___	___	___	pleasant

In relation to MYSELF:
MY CHOICES ARE

shrinking	___	___	___	___	___	___	___	expanding
seeking	___	___	___	___	___	___	___	avoiding
assertive	___	___	___	___	___	___	___	timid
important	___	___	___	___	___	___	___	unimportant
orderly	___	___	___	___	___	___	___	chaotic
intentional	___	___	___	___	___	___	___	unintentional
unpleasant	___	___	___	___	___	___	___	pleasant
constrained	___	___	___	___	___	___	___	free
worthless	___	___	___	___	___	___	___	valuable
following	___	___	___	___	___	___	___	leading
superficial	___	___	___	___	___	___	___	profound
informed	___	___	___	___	___	___	___	uninformed
timid	___	___	___	___	___	___	___	assertive

(Please go to NEXT PAGE and continue)

BARRETT PKPCT, Version I, PART 2

In relations with my FAMILY:
MY FREEDOM TO ACT INTENTIONALLY IS

timid	___ | ___ | ___ | ___ | ___ | ___ | ___	assertive
uninformed	___ | ___ | ___ | ___ | ___ | ___ | ___	informed
leading	___ | ___ | ___ | ___ | ___ | ___ | ___	following
profound	___ | ___ | ___ | ___ | ___ | ___ | ___	superficial
expanding	___ | ___ | ___ | ___ | ___ | ___ | ___	shrinking
unimportant	___ | ___ | ___ | ___ | ___ | ___ | ___	important
valuable	___ | ___ | ___ | ___ | ___ | ___ | ___	worthless
chaotic	___ | ___ | ___ | ___ | ___ | ___ | ___	orderly
avoiding	___ | ___ | ___ | ___ | ___ | ___ | ___	seeking
free	___ | ___ | ___ | ___ | ___ | ___ | ___	constrained
unintentional	___ | ___ | ___ | ___ | ___ | ___ | ___	intentional
pleasant	___ | ___ | ___ | ___ | ___ | ___ | ___	unpleasant
orderly	___ | ___ | ___ | ___ | ___ | ___ | ___	chaotic

In relations with my FAMILY:
MY INVOLVEMENT IN CREATING CHANGE IS

unintentional	___ | ___ | ___ | ___ | ___ | ___ | ___	intentional
expanding	___ | ___ | ___ | ___ | ___ | ___ | ___	shrinking
profound	___ | ___ | ___ | ___ | ___ | ___ | ___	superficial
chaotic	___ | ___ | ___ | ___ | ___ | ___ | ___	orderly
free	___ | ___ | ___ | ___ | ___ | ___ | ___	constrained
valuable	___ | ___ | ___ | ___ | ___ | ___ | ___	worthless
uninformed	___ | ___ | ___ | ___ | ___ | ___ | ___	informed
avoiding	___ | ___ | ___ | ___ | ___ | ___ | ___	seeking
leading	___ | ___ | ___ | ___ | ___ | ___ | ___	following
unimportant	___ | ___ | ___ | ___ | ___ | ___ | ___	important
timid	___ | ___ | ___ | ___ | ___ | ___ | ___	assertive
pleasant	___ | ___ | ___ | ___ | ___ | ___ | ___	unpleasant
superficial	___ | ___ | ___ | ___ | ___ | ___ | ___	profound

THANK YOU

INTRODUCTION TO BARRETT'S PKPCT

The PKPCT is designed to help you describe the meaning of day-to-day change in your life. Four indicators of experiencing change are:

> **AWARENESS**
> **CHOICES**
> **FREEDOM TO ACT INTENTIONALLY**
> **INVOLVEMENT IN CREATING CHANGE**

It takes about 10 minutes to complete the PKPCT.

INSTRUCTIONS FOR COMPLETING BARRETT'S PKPCT

For each indicator, there are 13 lines. There are words at both ends of each line. The meaning of the words are opposite to each other. There are 7 spaces between each pair of words which provide a range of possible responses. Place an "X" in the space along the line that best describes the meaning of the indicator (AWARENESS, CHOICES, FREEDOM TO ACT INTENTIONALLY, or INVOLVEMENT IN CREATING CHANGE) for you at this time.

For example:
Under the indicator CHOICES, if your CHOICES are quite closely described as "informed," your answer might look like this:

> informed ___|_X_|___|___|___|___|___ uninformed

If your CHOICES are quite closely described as "uninformed," your answer might look like this:

> informed ___|___|___|___|___|_X_|___ uninformed

If your CHOICES are equally "informed" and "uninformed," place an "X" in the middle space on the line. Your answer might look like this:

> informed ___|___|___|_X_|___|___|___ uninformed

REMEMBER:
- There are no right or wrong answers.
- Record your first impression for **each pair of words**.
- You can place an "X" in any space along the line that best describes the meaning the indicator has for you at this time.
- Mark only one "X" for each pair of words.
- Mark an "X" for every pair of words.

PLEASE BEGIN TO MARK YOUR X'S ON BARRETT'S PKPCT

 (Please go to NEXT PAGE and continue)

BARRETT PKPCT, Version II

MY AWARENESS IS

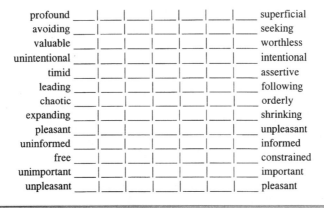

profound ___|___|___|___|___|___|___	superficial
avoiding ___|___|___|___|___|___|___	seeking
valuable ___|___|___|___|___|___|___	worthless
unintentional ___|___|___|___|___|___|___	intentional
timid ___|___|___|___|___|___|___	assertive
leading ___|___|___|___|___|___|___	following
chaotic ___|___|___|___|___|___|___	orderly
expanding ___|___|___|___|___|___|___	shrinking
pleasant ___|___|___|___|___|___|___	unpleasant
uninformed ___|___|___|___|___|___|___	informed
free ___|___|___|___|___|___|___	constrained
unimportant ___|___|___|___|___|___|___	important
unpleasant ___|___|___|___|___|___|___	pleasant

MY CHOICES ARE

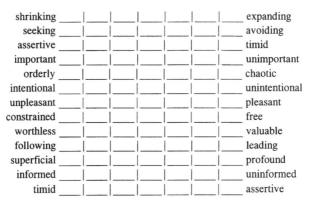

shrinking ___|___|___|___|___|___|___	expanding
seeking ___|___|___|___|___|___|___	avoiding
assertive ___|___|___|___|___|___|___	timid
important ___|___|___|___|___|___|___	unimportant
orderly ___|___|___|___|___|___|___	chaotic
intentional ___|___|___|___|___|___|___	unintentional
unpleasant ___|___|___|___|___|___|___	pleasant
constrained ___|___|___|___|___|___|___	free
worthless ___|___|___|___|___|___|___	valuable
following ___|___|___|___|___|___|___	leading
superficial ___|___|___|___|___|___|___	profound
informed ___|___|___|___|___|___|___	uninformed
timid ___|___|___|___|___|___|___	assertive

(Please go to NEXT PAGE and continue)

BARRETT PKPCT, Version II, PART 2

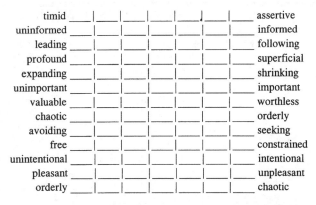

MY **FREEDOM TO ACT INTENTIONALLY** IS

timid	___	___	___	___	___	___	___	___	assertive
uninformed	___	___	___	___	___	___	___	___	informed
leading	___	___	___	___	___	___	___	___	following
profound	___	___	___	___	___	___	___	___	superficial
expanding	___	___	___	___	___	___	___	___	shrinking
unimportant	___	___	___	___	___	___	___	___	important
valuable	___	___	___	___	___	___	___	___	worthless
chaotic	___	___	___	___	___	___	___	___	orderly
avoiding	___	___	___	___	___	___	___	___	seeking
free	___	___	___	___	___	___	___	___	constrained
unintentional	___	___	___	___	___	___	___	___	intentional
pleasant	___	___	___	___	___	___	___	___	unpleasant
orderly	___	___	___	___	___	___	___	___	chaotic

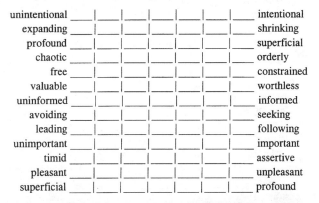

MY **INVOLVEMENT IN CREATING CHANGE** IS

unintentional	___	___	___	___	___	___	___	___	intentional
expanding	___	___	___	___	___	___	___	___	shrinking
profound	___	___	___	___	___	___	___	___	superficial
chaotic	___	___	___	___	___	___	___	___	orderly
free	___	___	___	___	___	___	___	___	constrained
valuable	___	___	___	___	___	___	___	___	worthless
uninformed	___	___	___	___	___	___	___	___	informed
avoiding	___	___	___	___	___	___	___	___	seeking
leading	___	___	___	___	___	___	___	___	following
unimportant	___	___	___	___	___	___	___	___	important
timid	___	___	___	___	___	___	___	___	assertive
pleasant	___	___	___	___	___	___	___	___	unpleasant
superficial	___	___	___	___	___	___	___	___	profound

THANK YOU

SCORING GUIDE

Scores are computed by assigning numbers from the scoring guide that correspond to participants' responses on the instrument.

BARRETT PKPCT, Version II

MARK AN "X" AS DESCRIBED IN THE INSTRUCTIONS

MY AWARENESS IS

	7	6	5	4	3	2	1	
profound	7	6	5	4	3	2	1	superficial
avoiding	1	2	3	4	5	6	7	seeking
valuable	7	6	5	4	3	2	1	worthless
unintentional	1	2	3	4	5	6	7	intentional
timid	1	2	3	4	5	6	7	assertive
leading	7	6	5	4	3	2	1	following
chaotic	1	2	3	4	5	6	7	orderly
expanding	7	6	5	4	3	2	1	shrinking
pleasant	7	6	5	4	3	2	1	unpleasant
uninformed	1	2	3	4	5	6	7	informed
free	7	6	5	4	3	2	1	constrained
unimportant	1	2	3	4	5	6	7	important
unpleasant	1	2	3	4	5	6	7	pleasant

MARK AN "X" AS DESCRIBED IN THE INSTRUCTIONS

MY CHOICES ARE

	1	2	3	4	5	6	7	
shrinking	1	2	3	4	5	6	7	expanding
seeking	7	6	5	4	3	2	1	avoiding
assertive	7	6	5	4	3	2	1	timid
important	7	6	5	4	3	2	1	unimportant
orderly	7	6	5	4	3	2	1	chaotic
intentional	7	6	5	4	3	2	1	unintentional
unpleasant	1	2	3	4	5	6	7	pleasant
constrained	1	2	3	4	5	6	7	free
worthless	1	2	3	4	5	6	7	valuable
following	1	2	3	4	5	6	7	leading
superficial	1	2	3	4	5	6	7	profound
informed	7	6	5	4	3	2	1	uninformed
timid	1	2	3	4	5	6	7	assertive

BARRETT PKPCT, Version II, PART 2

MARK AN "X" AS DESCRIBED IN THE INSTRUCTIONS

MY FREEDOM TO ACT INTENTIONALLY IS

	1	2	3	4	5	6	7	
timid	1	2	3	4	5	6	7	assertive
uninformed	1	2	3	4	5	6	7	informed
leading	7	6	5	4	3	2	1	following
profound	7	6	5	4	3	2	1	superficial
expanding	7	6	5	4	3	2	1	shrinking
unimportant	1	2	3	4	5	6	7	important
valuable	7	6	5	4	3	2	1	worthless
chaotic	1	2	3	4	5	6	7	orderly
avoiding	1	2	3	4	5	6	7	seeking
free	7	6	5	4	3	2	1	constrained
unintentional	1	2	3	4	5	6	7	intentional
pleasant	7	6	5	4	3	2	1	unpleasant
orderly	7	6	5	4	3	2	1	chaotic

MARK AN "X" AS DESCRIBED IN THE INSTRUCTIONS

MY INVOLVEMENT IN CREATING CHANGE IS

	1	2	3	4	5	6	7	
unintentional	1	2	3	4	5	6	7	intentional
expanding	7	6	5	4	3	2	1	shrinking
profound	7	6	5	4	3	2	1	superficial
chaotic	1	2	3	4	5	6	7	orderly
free	7	6	5	4	3	2	1	constrained
valuable	7	6	5	4	3	2	1	worthless
uninformed	1	2	3	4	5	6	7	informed
avoiding	1	2	3	4	5	6	7	seeking
leading	7	6	5	4	3	2	1	following
unimportant	1	2	3	4	5	6	7	important
timid	1	2	3	4	5	6	7	assertive
pleasant	7	6	5	4	3	2	1	unpleasant
superficial	1	2	3	4	5	6	7	profound

THANK YOU

BARRETT PKPCT, Version II

MARK AN "X" AS DESCRIBED IN THE INSTRUCTIONS

MY AWARENESS IS

Left	1	2	3	4	5	6	7	Right	
profound	X							superficial	6
avoiding		X						seeking	3
valuable			X					worthless	4
unintentional			X					intentional	4
timid		X						assertive	3
leading				X				following	3
chaotic					X			orderly	6
expanding						X		shrinking	1
pleasant					X			unpleasant	2
uninformed					X			informed	6
free				X				constrained	3
unimportant		X						important	$\frac{3}{2}$ (44)
unpleasant	X							pleasant	

MARK AN "X" AS DESCRIBED IN THE INSTRUCTIONS

MY CHOICES ARE

Left	1	2	3	4	5	6	7	Right	
shrinking	X							expanding	2
seeking		X						avoiding	5
assertive			X					timid	4
important		X						unimportant	5
orderly	X							chaotic	6
intentional	X							unintentional	7
unpleasant			X					pleasant	4
constrained						X		free	6
worthless							X	valuable	7
following					X			leading	5
superficial		X						profound	3
informed			X					uninformed	$\frac{4}{3}$ (58)
timid		X						assertive	3

BARRETT PKPCT, Version II, PART 2

MARK AN "X" AS DESCRIBED IN THE INSTRUCTIONS

MY FREEDOM TO ACT INTENTIONALLY IS

	1	2	3	4	5	6	7		
timid		x						assertive	2
uninformed			x					informed	3
leading				x				following	4
profound					x			superficial	3
expanding						x		shrinking	1
unimportant				x				important	4
valuable					x			worthless	3
chaotic						x		orderly	6
avoiding					x			seeking	5
free				x				constrained	4
unintentional		x						intentional	2
pleasant				x				unpleasant	4
orderly		x						chaotic	6

(41)

MARK AN "X" AS DESCRIBED IN THE INSTRUCTIONS

MY INVOLVEMENT IN CREATING CHANGE IS

	1	2	3	4	5	6	7		
unintentional							x	intentional	7
expanding						x		shrinking	2
profound					x			superficial	3
chaotic			x					orderly	4
free					x			constrained	3
valuable			x					worthless	4
uninformed		x						informed	3
avoiding			x					seeking	4
leading		x						following	5
unimportant		x						important	3
timid		x						assertive	3
pleasant						x		unpleasant	2
superficial	x							profound	2

(43)

THANK YOU

4

The Epilepsy Self-Efficacy Scale

Colleen DiIorio and Kate Yeager

This chapter discusses the Epilepsy Self-Efficacy Scale, a measure of a person's confidence in managing various aspects of an epilepsy self-management regimen.

PURPOSE

About 2 million people in the United States are diagnosed with epilepsy or seizure disorders. Most people with epilepsy must take prescribed medication to control their seizures. In addition, people who have seizures must develop certain strategies and behaviors to prevent a seizure occurrence or to reduce the impact of a seizure to themselves and others. Current estimates are that about 20% to 70% of persons taking medications for seizures do not always take them as prescribed, thus increasing their risk of having a seizure and the negative outcomes associated with seizures. In addition, not all people follow safety instructions or avoid things that might precipitate a seizure. Considerable research has been conducted to understand factors associated with medication adherence among people with epilepsy. These studies generally show that although medication adherence is a problem that equally affects men and women of all ages, ethnic backgrounds, and income levels, the complexity of the regimen and certain beliefs and attitudes about taking medications are important in understanding adherence. Self-efficacy is one belief that has emerged from the literature on chronic illness as a factor in understanding adherence to long-term regimens.

CONCEPTUAL FRAMEWORK

Social cognitive theory served as the conceptual framework for the development of the Epilepsy Self-Efficacy Scale (ESES). Bandura (1997), the progenitor of the theory, proposes a dynamic interplay among the person, the environment, and behavior, and that this interplay determines what behaviors a person chooses to perform and his or her level of perseverance. The most salient personal factor endorsed by the theory is that of self-efficacy. Bandura (1997) defines self-efficacy as "beliefs in one's capabilities to organize and execute the courses of action required to produce given attainments" (p. 3). Research has demonstrated that people who hold strong beliefs about their self-efficacy with respect to a selected behavior are more likely to attempt to perform that behavior and to persevere until they have mastered the behavior.

Efficacy beliefs vary in magnitude, strength, and generality (Bandura, 1997). Magnitude refers to the perceived level of difficulty of a particular behavior. Behaviors may be relatively easy under some conditions but perceived as more difficult under other conditions. For example, a person may find that taking one pill once or even twice a day is relatively easy, but taking a pill three or more times a day is much more difficult to do. Strength refers to the degree of confidence a person has in his or her ability to perform a given behavior. The strength of one's efficacy beliefs is generally assessed by asking people to evaluate their degree of confidence on a rating scale from *not at all certain I can do* to *very certain I can do*. Finally, generality refers to the generalizability of efficacy beliefs from one behavior to another. For example, confidence in being able to take epilepsy medications may generalize to confidence in taking any medications on a regular basis.

Bandura (1997) cautions that because people have varying levels of confidence regarding their performance on a variety of behaviors, it is impossible to measure a general construct of self-efficacy that could be used to assess perceived efficacy for the performance of all behaviors. Thus, he endorses the use of behavior-specific self-efficacy measures. To measure self-efficacy for the performance of behaviors important in the self-management of epilepsy, an instrument with items specific to the tasks associated with epilepsy self-management is necessary. For the development of the instrument, epilepsy self-efficacy was defined as a person's belief in the ability to manage his or her epilepsy (seizure condition). Three dimensions of epilepsy self-efficacy were identified: medication management, seizure management, and general management.

PROCEDURES FOR THE DEVELOPMENT OF THE ESES

Items for the ESES were derived from a review of the literature on epilepsy and self-efficacy, a review of existing self-efficacy scales, a review of educational materials for people with epilepsy, and discussions with health care professionals and people with epilepsy. Thirty-four items representing the three dimensions of medication management, seizure management, and general management were written. This first set of items was reviewed for clarity, readability, meaning, and unidimensionality by a group of physicians, nurses, and people with epilepsy. Based on their comments, changes were made in the wording of items to improve clarity.

Content validity was assessed using procedures described by Waltz, Strickland, and Lenz (1991). In the first phase of this process, four experts in epilepsy and self-efficacy were asked to evaluate each of the 34 items and rate each item as to its degree of relevancy to the concept of epilepsy self-efficacy. The experts made several suggestions for changes in the wording of the items, and Bandura, one of the expert judges suggested changing the rating scale from a 5- to an 11-point scale. He also suggested that the word *always* be included in each item so as to reduce the tendency to rate each item at the highest level of agreement. Items that did not adequately address the concept of epilepsy self-efficacy were deleted, yielding a 28-item instrument. Following these changes, a panel of persons with epilepsy reviewed the ESES. They were asked to review each item for clarity, readability, and correspondence with their experience. Following their review and minor changes in the items, the four members of the expert panel were asked again to review the revised instrument. They again rated each item as to its degree of relevancy to the concept of epilepsy self-efficacy using a 4-point rating scale, with a score of 1 indicating *not at all relevant* and a score of 4 indicating *very relevant* to the concept of epilepsy self-efficacy. A content validity index (CVI) was computed using procedures described by Waltz et al. (1991) and was 94%, indicating a high level of agreement among the judges that the items measured the concept of epilepsy self-efficacy.

An item analysis was conducted using data obtained from a study of epilepsy self-management. Data were obtained from questionnaires completed by 98 participants in a job-training program offered by a local epilepsy foundation. A review of interitem correlations revealed that the correlation between two items was .84, suggesting redundancy of content. After reviewing these items, one item was deleted. A review of the item-to-total scale correlations showed that three items failed to meet the criterion value for correlation with the total scale. That is, the item-to-total correlation for each of these items was less than .30, as suggested by Nunnally & Bernstein (1994). One item was reworded, and the other two items were deleted. With the deletion of three items, the 1992 version of the ESES consisted of 25 items (ESES-92). In 2000, eight items were added to the ESES in an effort to more fully assess the general management aspect of epilepsy self-management (see Appendix).

DESCRIPTION OF THE ESES

The ESES-92 is a 25-item self-report scale assessing a person's belief in his or her ability to carry out tasks associated with epilepsy self-management. The items represent three dimensions of self-management: medication management, seizure management, and general management, including safety and health. Respondents are asked to rate each item on an 11-point scale from

0 (*I cannot do at all*) to 100 (*Sure I can do*). Above the midpoint of 50 is written the words *Moderately sure I can do*. Respondents are instructed to rate their level of confidence if they were asked to do the tasks today. All items are positively worded. There are 14 items representing medication management. An example of an item representing this dimension is "I can always plan ahead so that I do not run out of seizure medication." Eight items were written to assess seizure management. An example of an item addressing seizure management is "I can always take care of the day-to-day changes in my epilepsy." Three items assess general management, and an example of an item representing this dimension is "I can always handle situations that upset me." The 2000 version (ESES-2000) has an additional 8 items that address general management issues, such as stress management, exercise, and diet. The ESES has been translated into Thai and Hebrew. For the Thai version items number 2, 9 and 21 were deleted and six new items were added (Table 4.1). The scale was first translated into Thai, and then translated back into English.

ADMINISTRATION AND SCORING OF THE ESES

The ESES is a self-report measure and can be administered in several ways. In one study, trained interviewers administered the instrument to participants as part of an in-person interview. In this study, the interviewers read each item to the participants and recorded their answers. In another study, participants completed their own survey. In this study, a trained interviewer assisted participants who had difficulty reading. The ESES has also been administered as part of a mail-out survey conducted among people who were enrolled in a job-training program.

In a recent study, the ESES has been included in a computer-based battery of assessments. In this project, participants respond to items read to them using computer technology. The items also appear on the screen so that a person can read and hear each item. The respondent then selects his or her response on the screen using a stylus. To move to the next question, the respondent selects a *next question* box.

Responses to each item on the scale are summed to yield a total score. Total scores range from 0 to 2,500 (25 items in ESES-92) or to 3,300 (33 items in ESES-2000). Because of the large range of total scores, an alternative approach to scoring is to obtain a mean item score. This score can be obtained by dividing the total score by the number of items answered. In this latter case, total scores range from 0 to 100. In both scoring methods higher scores represent a high degree of self-efficacy in epilepsy self-management.

RELIABILITY AND VALIDITY

Table 4.1 presents information on reliability and validity testing.

TABLE 4.1 Reliability and Validity Studies for the Epilepsy Self-Efficacy Scale.

Study citation	Sample and characteristics	Reliability evidence	Validity evidence
DiIorio, Faherty, & Manteuffel (1992)	Sample 1: 12 Sample 2: 28 Sample 3: 98 *Sample characteristics:* Sample 1: Mean age = 33.8; 9 male, 3 female; 7 White Sample 2: Mean age = 35.6; 53.3% male; 72.4% White Sample 3: Mean age = 35.5; 52% female; 73.5% White	*Test-retest:* .81 over a 4-week period *Internal consistency:* Sample 2: Cronbach's alpha = .91 Sample 3: Cronbach's alpha = .93 Interitem correlation: Range −.01 to .89 Item-to total correlations— Range .23 to .72	*A priori content validity:* Review of epilepsy and self-efficacy literature, existing self-efficacy scales, epilepsy educational materials, and discussions with health care professionals and people with epilepsy *Posteriori content validity:* Panel of four experts in epilepsy and self-efficacy CVI = 94% *Construct validity:* Relationship in the predicted direction between ESES and a measure of epilepsy self-management (r = .50) and between ESES and a measure of social support (r = .48).
DiIorio, Faherty, & Manteuffel (1993)	*Sample size:* 98 *Sample characteristics:* Mean age = 35.5; 52% female; 73.5% White	*Internal consistency:* Cronbach's alpha = .93	*Construct validity:* Relationship in the predicted direction between ESES and a measure of epilepsy self-

TABLE 4.1 (*continued*)

Study citation	Sample and characteristics	Reliability evidence	Validity evidence
DiIorio, Faherty, & Manteuffel (1993) (*continued*)			management ($r = .50$) and between ESES and a measure of social support ($r = .48$). Same data as reported above on sample 3.
DiIorio, Faherty, & Manteuffel (1994)	*Sample size:* 80 *Sample characteristics:* Mean age = 38.2; 54% male; 73.7% White, 26.2% Black	*Internal consistency:* Cronbach's alpha = .94	*Construct validity:* Relationship in the predicted direction between ESES and a measure of epilepsy self-management ($r = .44$), between ESES and a measure of social support ($r = .38$), and between ESES and a measure of self-esteem ($r = .38$).
DiIorio, Hennessy, & Manteuffel (1996)	*Sample size:* 195 *Sample characteristics:* Mean age = 35.8; 58.5% female; 69.7% White, 27.1% Black		*Construct validity:* Through structural equation modeling, self-efficacy was positively related to outcome expectancy and negatively related to anxiety.

TABLE 4.1 (*continued*)

Study citation	Sample and characteristics	Reliability evidence	Validity evidence
Amir, Roziner, Knoll, & Neufeld (1999)	*Sample size:* 89 *Sample characteristics:* Mean age = 35.7; 58% male	*Internal consistency:* Cronbach's alpha = .94 ESES translated into Hebrew for this study	*Construct validity:* Relationship in the predicted direction between ESES and a measure of seizure severity (percept; $r = .50$ and ictal, $r = .52$), between ESES and a measure of social support ($r = .53$), between ESES and a measure of locus of control ($r = .58$), and between ESES and a measure of quality of life ($r = .61$).
DiIorio et al. (in progress)	*Sample size:* 160 *Sample characteristics:* Mean age = 40.9; 4.6% male; 85.9% White, 9.0% Black	*Internal consistency:* 33-item measure Cronbach's alpha = .89	*Construct validity: Preliminary Data:* Relationship in the predicted direction between ESES and a measure of depression ($r = .43$), between ESES and a measure of social support ($r = .35$), between ESES and a measure of self-management ($r = .26$), between ESES and a measure of 3 types of outcome expectancies ($r = .40, .37, .19$),

TABLE 4.1 *(continued)*

Study citation	Sample and characteristics	Reliability evidence	Validity evidence
DiIorio et al. (in progress) *(continued)*			and between ESES and a measure of patient satisfaction ($r = .27$).
S. Niyomkai (personal communication, 2001)	*Sample size:* 20 *Sample characteristics:* Age range = 13–21	*Internal consistency:* Cronbach's alpha = .86 Deleted 3 items due to cultural issues. Added 6 new items to increase measures of general lifestyle: 1. I can always choose the food that can nourish and make me strong. 2. I can always avoid alcoholic beverages that can worsen the disease. 3. I can always do exercises that are appropriate to me. 4. I can always know when to quit exercise. 5. I can always keep myself from feeling lonely. 6. I am confident that I am strong enough to stand the disease.	None.

CONCLUSIONS AND RECOMMENDATIONS

The ESES was developed to measure a person's level of confidence in carrying out tasks associated with epilepsy self-management. Reliability and validity assessments conducted thus far indicate that the ESES meets the standards for a reliable and valid measure of epilepsy self-efficacy. Cronbach's alpha coefficients have ranged from .86 to .94, indicating adequate internal consistency for a new instrument. Test-retest reliability demonstrated fair consistency over a 4-week period. Moreover, the ESES has correlated in the predicted directions with measures of the theoretically meaningful constructs of epilepsy self-management, social support, quality of life, outcome expectancies, and anxiety supporting the validity of the measure. Factor analysis revealed two factors whose items did not always correspond with the three preconceived dimensions. These results suggest that the underlying structure of the ESES is more complex than originally conceptualized.

Because the sample for the assessment of test-retest reliability was relatively small, a greater number of participants should be recruited to reassess the stability of the ESES over time. The items for the ESES were selected based on three predetermined content areas of medication management, seizure management, and general management. Because the results of a factor analysis revealed that the items did not correspond completely with three preconceived dimensions, further analysis with a sample size of at least 300 individuals is required to examine more closely the stability of the factors and the underlying structure of the scale. Analyses using item response approaches will be helpful in identifying items that are most useful for the measure of epilepsy self-efficacy.

Thus far, the psychometric analyses of the scale have been conducted using responses from samples of predominantly White participants. Further study is necessary to determine the usefulness of the scale for members of other races and cultures.

ACKNOWLEDGMENTS

Some data from this chapter were published in previous journal reports appearing in Journal of Neuroscience Nursing, Western Journal of Nursing Research, Research in Nursing and Health, and Nursing Research. Funded by NINR Grant R01NR-04770.

REFERENCES

Amir, A., Roziner, I., Knoll, A., & Neufeld, M. (1999). Self-efficacy and social support as mediators in the relation between disease severity and quality of life in patients with epilepsy. *Epilepsia, 40,* 216–224.

Bandura, A. (1997). *Self-efficacy: The exercise of control.* New York: W. H. Freeman.

DiIorio, C., Faherty, B., & Manteuffel, B. (1992). The development and testing of an instrument to measure self-efficacy in individuals with epilepsy. *Journal of Neuroscience Nursing, 24,* 9–13.

DiIorio, C., Faherty, B., & Manteuffel, B. (1993). Self-efficacy and social support in self-management of epilepsy. *Western Journal of Nursing Research, 14,* 292–307.

DiIorio, C., Faherty, B., & Manteuffel, B. (1994). Epilepsy self- management: Partial replication and extension. *Research in Nursing and Health, 17,* 167–174.

DiIorio, C., Hennessy, M., & Manteuffel, B. (1996). Epilepsy self- management: A test of a theoretical model. *Nursing Research 45,* 211–217.

DiIorio, C., Shafer, P., Letz, R., Henry, T., Schomer, D., & Yeager, K. (in progress). *A test of an epilepsy self management model.*

Nunnally, J., & Bernstein, I. (1994). *Psychometric theory* (3rd ed.). New York: McGraw-Hill.

Waltz, C., Strickland, O., & Lenz, E. (1991). *Measurement in nursing research.* Philadelphia: F. A. Davis.

APPENDIX: EPILEPSY SELF-EFFICACY

	I cannot do at all					Moderately sure I can do					Sure I can do
1. I can always take my seizure medication when I am away from home.	0	1	2	3	4	5	6	7	8	9	10
2. I can stay on my seizure medication most of the time.	0	1	2	3	4	5	6	7	8	9	10
*3. I can always practice relaxation exercises to help me manage stress.	0	1	2	3	4	5	6	7	8	9	10
4. I can always name my seizure medication.	0	1	2	3	4	5	6	7	8	9	10
5. I can always plan ahead so that I do not run out of my seizure medication.	0	1	2	3	4	5	6	7	8	9	10
*6. I can always get enough exercise.	0	1	2	3	4	5	6	7	8	9	10
7. I can always take my seizure medication on holidays, birthdays, vacations, and other special occasions.	0	1	2	3	4	5	6	7	8	9	10
8. I can have fun with other people and still manage my epilepsy.	0	1	2	3	4	5	6	7	8	9	10
9. I can always take my seizure medication around people who do not know that I have seizures.	0	1	2	3	4	5	6	7	8	9	10
*10. I can always use stress management techniques to stop seizures.	0	1	2	3	4	5	6	7	8	9	10
11. I can always take care of day-to-day changes in my epilepsy.	0	1	2	3	4	5	6	7	8	9	10
12. I can always manage my epilepsy in new situations.	0	1	2	3	4	5	6	7	8	9	10
13. I can always tell when I am having side effects from my seizure medication.	0	1	2	3	4	5	6	7	8	9	10
*14. I can always eat healthy meals.	0	1	2	3	4	5	6	7	8	9	10
15. I can always deal with any side effects from my seizure medication.	0	1	2	3	4	5	6	7	8	9	10
16. I can always manage my epilepsy.	0	1	2	3	4	5	6	7	8	9	10
*17. I can always recognize situations or activities that may make my seizures worse.	0	1	2	3	4	5	6	7	8	9	10
18. I can always find ways to get enough sleep.	0	1	2	3	4	5	6	7	8	9	10
19. I can always handle situations that upset me.	0	1	2	3	4	5	6	7	8	9	10
20. I can always fit my seizure medication schedule around my daily activities.	0	1	2	3	4	5	6	7	8	9	10
21. I can always do what needs to be done if I miss a dose of my seizure medication.	0	1	2	3	4	5	6	7	8	9	10

APPENDIX: *(continued)*

	I cannot do at all				Moderately sure I can do					Sure I can do	
*22. I can always find ways to do things that I enjoy to help me manage stress.	0	1	2	3	4	5	6	7	8	9	10
23. I can always follow my seizure medication schedule.	0	1	2	3	4	5	6	7	8	9	10
24. I can always call my doctor or nurse when I need to ask a question or report a seizure.	0	1	2	3	4	5	6	7	8	9	10
25. I can always keep my epilepsy under control.	0	1	2	3	4	5	6	7	8	9	10
26. I can always take time out from my daily activities to go to the doctor for an epilepsy checkup.	0	1	2	3	4	5	6	7	8	9	10
*27. I can always avoid situations or activities that make my seizures worse.	0	1	2	3	4	5	6	7	8	9	10
28. I can always drive or get a ride to the doctor's office when I need to see him or her.	0	1	2	3	4	5	6	7	8	9	10
29. I can always get medical help when needed for my seizures.	0	1	2	3	4	5	6	7	8	9	10
30. I can always find ways to remember to take my seizure medication.	0	1	2	3	4	5	6	7	8	9	10
*31. I always carry personal identification in case I have a seizure.	0	1	2	3	4	5	6	7	8	9	10
32. I can always find a way to get seizure medication if I go out of town and forget mine.	0	1	2	3	4	5	6	7	8	9	10
33. I can always get my seizure medication refilled when I need to.	0	1	2	3	4	5	6	7	8	9	10

*Items added for ESES 2000.

51

5

The Insulin Management Diabetes Self-Efficacy Scale

Ann C. Hurley and Rose M. Harvey

This chapter discusses the Insulin Management Diabetes Self-Efficacy Scale, a measure of individuals' beliefs in their ability to organize and carry out their diabetes self-care plan.

PURPOSE

The Insulin Management Diabetes Self-Efficacy Scale (IMDSES) was designed to be used as an assessment guide to identify individuals who might benefit from individual and group confidence-building exercises designed to complement traditional diabetes health education. The IMDSES may also be used as an outcome measure to identify specific areas in the diabetes regimen where an individual needs help or to evaluate the effectiveness of a diabetes education program.

CONCEPTUAL BASIS

Self-efficacy (Bandura, 1977) refers to personal beliefs of how well one can organize and carry out patterns of behavior that may contain novel, unpredictable, and stressful elements (Bandura, 1982). Bandura (1986) suggests that self-efficacy is a powerful psychosocial variable capable of predicting the enactment of health-related behaviors.

A literature review of the first decade of self-efficacy and health behavior research found that high levels of self-efficacy were positively associated with carrying out regimen-specific behaviors (O'Leary, 1985). Because the regimen required to control diabetes requires that individuals plan and carry out actions in diverse circumstances and settings, there is a pragmatic interconnection between perceived self-efficacy and self-care of diabetes mellitus. To test this relationship, two diabetes scales were developed to make self-efficacy operational. Crabtree (1986) developed a scale to measure diabetes self-efficacy in adults and found that diabetes self-efficacy predicted diabetes behaviors of adults who self-managed their disorder. Grossman, Brink, and Hauser (1987) developed a scale for use with children and found that self-efficacy of adolescent girls was correlated with their metabolic state.

In the past decade, a number of research studies have provided additional empirical support for the relationship between diabetes self-efficacy and diabetes self-care. Adolescents who reported lower adherence also reported lower self-efficacy (Littlefield et al., 1992). In 118 inner-city African American women, level of self-efficacy explained diet, exercise, and home-testing behaviors (Skelly, Marshall, Haughey, Davis, & Dunford, 1995). A study of 149 patients with insulin-dependent diabetes found that perception of self-efficacy may be a common behavioral factor determining both diabetes self-care and oral health behavior (Kneckt, Syrjala, Laukkanen, & Knuuttila, 1999). Examination of a motivational theory of diabetes self-care that postulated links between self-efficacy and autonomous self-regulation using constraint analysis found that self-efficacy was related to adherence, and autonomous self-regulation was associated with life satisfaction (Senecal, Nouwen, & White, 2000).

Bernal, Wooley, Schensul, and Dickinson (2000) used the Spanish-language translation of the IMDSES reported in this chapter to examine self-efficacy and self-care in a sample of 97 insulin-requiring adults. They found that: (1) behaviors that required problem solving in changing circumstances received the lowest scores, (2) attending diabetes classes and having home nursing visits were associated with an increased sense of efficacy, particularly in the areas of diet and insulin management; and (3) English speaking was associated with a general sense of self-efficacy in managing diabetes care.

Additionally, many articles have suggested that diabetes self-efficacy be included in educational programs for both patients and providers. Glasgow and Osteen (1992) have long suggested that the evaluation of diabetes education should include measures of self-efficacy. Self-efficacy is suggested as a framework for the development of community pharmacy-based diabetes education programs (Johnson, 1996). Self-efficacy was also used with third-year medical students as an outcome measure of a computer-assisted diabetes nutrition program (Engel, Crandall, Basch, Zybert, & Wylie-Rosett, 1997). A research-based article on diabetes care concluded that "boosting a person's judgement of his or her ability to perform specific diabetes activities is an important step toward improving self-care" (Corbett, 1999, p. 594). Lorenz, Gregory, and Davis (2000) suggest that self-efficacy be used in educating professional providers in diabetes care. They found that post-training self-efficacy for meeting educational objectives increased after training and correlated with reported successful practice. As a result, Lorenz and colleagues suggested that self-efficacy assessments can contribute to clinical training program evaluation. Day (2000) agreed and stated that education in the learning process, including psychosocial factors governing behavior (i.e., self-efficacy), is essential for all clinicians involved in providing patient care and especially to promote success in managing diabetes mellitus.

Definitions

Self-efficacy is a sense of "I can do." "Perceived self-efficacy refers to beliefs in one's capabilities to organize and execute courses of action required to meet given situational demands" (Bandura, 1986, p. 391). Self-efficacy means individuals' judgments of their capability to monitor, plan, and carry out their diabetes activities of daily living. Self-efficacy is a concept that is oriented to behaviors, and as such it is concerned with the actions that people take rather than the outcomes that are expected to follow.

The self-efficacy concept has three dimensions: magnitude, strength, and generality. Each dimension was clearly distinct in the scales used for the initial phobic research series conducted by Bandura and colleagues (Bandura & Adams, 1977; Bandura, Adams, & Beyer, 1977; Bandura, Adams, Hurdy, & Howell, 1980; Bandura, Reese, & Adams, 1982). The cluster of smoking investigations (Coelho, 1984; Colletti, Supnick, & Payne, 1985; Condiotte & Lichtenstein, 1981; DiClemente, 1981; DiClemente, Prochaska, & Gibertini, 1985; McIntyre, Lichtenstein, & Mermelstein, 1983; Prochaska, Crimi, Lapsanski, Martel, & Reid, 1982) that followed the phobic studies combined the three dimensions in the measures used to make smoking self-efficacy operational. Crabtree (1986) had selected this latter format for the Diabetes Self-Efficacy Scale (DSES). Therefore, the IMDSES, building on the DSES, was also developed in the same format.

PROCEDURES FOR DEVELOPMENT

The Crabtree (1986) DSES was developed to be used with adults who have diabetes, regardless of the type of diabetes or of whether or not individuals used insulin. With both the permission and advice of Dr. Crabtree, the IMDSES was developed from the DSES and modified for adults who use insulin. The IMDSES measures individuals' confidence in their capacity to plan, carry out, monitor, make decisions about their self-care management plan, and adjust their diabetes activities of daily living accordingly.

The Crabtree 32-item DSES had been constructed with advice from Dr. Bandura and tested with a sample of 48 adults. For the IMDSES, a scale development blueprint for writing new items and revising some of the Crabtree (1986) items was developed so that individuals would interpret the statements as being specific to their diabetes activities of daily living.

Items were constructed to reflect only the self-efficacy concept and not related concepts, such as locus of control or self-esteem. Other item characteristics were that (1) the action word was an act, not an outcome; (2) items contained only one behavior; (3) "1 can" or a negative wording of "I can" was used to anchor the assertion in the present; (4) the word *diabetic* was used as an adjective, not a noun; (5) circumstances to reflect different situations, such as daily tedium or feeling sick, were used; and (6) the word *insulin* replaced the generic term *medication*. Sample items are "I can stay on my diabetic diet when I eat in unfamiliar places" and "I'm not sure I can recognize when my blood sugar is low."

The 26-item IMDSES (2 items are retained in the administration of the scale but are not used in scoring the IMDSES) was developed within a norm-referenced framework to test for varying levels of efficacy. Seven types of diabetes behaviors were represented: (1) general, (2) diet, (3) exercise, (4) foot care, (5) monitoring, (6) insulin administration, and (7) detecting, preventing, or treating high and low blood glucose reactions. Four general items were placed at the beginning and two at the end of the scale. The other items were arranged in similar clusters in a sequence determined by the diabetes content experts. Ten items were randomly selected to be worded negatively.

ADMINISTRATION AND SCORING

Efficacy assertions are made privately to avoid the possible influence of public disclosure on the target behavior (Telch, Bandura, Vinciguerra, Agras, & Stout, 1982). The IMDSES is a paper-and-pencil test with items and response selection on a Likert scale ranging from 1 (*strongly agree*) to 6 (*strongly disagree*). A "not applicable" category is provided and was coded as missing data for computing measurement reliability estimates (see Appendix). The 18 positively worded items are reverse-scored, so higher scores are interpreted as meaning the individual tested has a higher level of self-efficacy. Mean scores of items, subscales, and the scale total range from 1 (lowest) to 6 (highest). The IMDSES scale total score (range 26–156) or the three subscales—general, Diet, and Insulin—can be used. There are only two items on foot care and two items on exercise, and this small a number precludes having subscales for those behaviors.

A sequence of steps was followed to examine and adjust the IMDSES to ensure that the scale would have adequate psychometric properties. The initial DSES, developed with the advice of content specialists and using the results of three phases of' empirical testing, was considered to be a reliable and valid new instrument (Crabtree, 1986).

The IMDSES used some of the DSES items, but others were slightly modified to be consistent with the table of specifications. The *Diabetes Teaching Guide* (Joslin Diabetes Center, 1986) provided the diabetes content domain for additional items. Three diabetes educator nurses served as content specialists, and five patients reviewed and edited the items for understanding and clarity from the users' viewpoints. Six self-efficacy judges then rated the items for conceptual distinction, relevance, and clarity. Level of agreement provided quantification that a content validity index beyond the .05 level of significance had been achieved (Lynn, 1986). Finally, two phases of empirical testing provided evidence of reliability by test stability, internal consistency, preliminary factor structure, and convergent validity.

Sample and Setting

Initial empirical testing was conducted in two phases. First, an outpatient sample of 38 participants from a diabetes clinic provided data for the reliability estimates, of whom 27 participated in the retest phases. Second, an inpatient sample from a diabetes center located in the same large metropolitan New England city provided additional data for computing reliability estimates. This combined sample of 127 participants (38 outpatients and 89 inpatients) provided evidence for convergent validity and preliminary factor structure.

The IMDSES was refined on the basis of data from a second inpatient sample ($n = 142$). This phase allowed hypothesis testing of self-efficacy beliefs prior to discharge with self-care management reported 1 month later and microanalysis of the relationships between IMDSES subscales and related self-care practices.

Participant inclusion criteria were (1) diagnosis of diabetes mellitus; (2) use of insulin; (3) followed by Diabetes Center; (4) free of serious disorders and debilitating diabetic sequelae (blindness, marked neuropathy, incapacitating renal or cardiovascular problems); (5) in a nonacute phase of diabetes (not in acidosis or initiating hemodialysis); (6) not on nor planning to begin use of an insulin infusion pump in the next month; (7) no known mental impairment and presence of English-language skills, reading, and cognitive capacities to participate in the investigation; (8) 18 to 73 years of age; (9) not known to be pregnant; (10) not recommended for exclusion by nurse or physician; and (11) be willing to provide informed consent.

There were no statistically significant differences in the demographic variables or diabetes characteristics between the outpatient participants who participated in the retest phase ($n = 27$) and those who did not ($n = 11$) or between the inpatients who participated in initial testing (127) and hypothesis testing (142). The combined sample of outpatient participants ($n = 38$) was similar to the sample of inpatient participants ($n = 89$) except that outpatients were older ($M = 47.92$), $t(124) = 2.43$, $p < .017$) than the inpatients ($M = 40.28$). The demographic and diabetes characteristics of the combined data set ($N = 127$) in the initial empirical testing were used to describe the sample.

Participants were middle-aged and had many years of experience in self-care management of their diabetes. The average duration of diagnosed diabetes was 12 years ($SD = 8.1$), and participants had required insulin for 10.2 years ($SD = 8.3$). More females ($n = 71$) than males ($n = 56$) participated in the study. Most participants were married ($n = 75$). More participants lived with someone else ($n = 109$), such as parents ($n = 19$), spouse or one good adult friend ($n = 48$), or one adult and a child or children ($n = 42$) than lived alone ($n = 17$). The sample was considered well educated. Only seven participants had less than a high school education, the most common educational level of the majority ($n = 47$). Other participants had a postsecondary technical or vocational education ($n = 19$), college or university degree ($n = 33$), or graduate degree ($n = 16$). The majority ($n = 75$) were out of the house for over 40 hours a week holding a full-time job or were volunteers or full-time students. Participants were employed in a variety of positions that were categorized as professional ($n = 20$), technical ($n = 12$), clerical ($n = 20$), laborer ($n = 8$), or supervisor ($n = 6$). The remaining participants were at home ($n = 34$) or were full-time students ($n = 12$), or data were missing ($n = 15$).

In general, most participants had complex diabetes regimens that they were required to manage. Sixty-nine percent of the sample required two daily injections of insulin to control their diabetes. The number and type of daily insulin injections were as follows: (1) one daily injection of a single type of insulin ($n = 25$); (2) one daily injection and two types of insulin ($n = 14$); (3) two daily injections, each with a single type of insulin ($n = 16$); (4) two daily injections: one with a single insulin and one with two types of insulin ($n = 17$); (5) two daily injections of two types of insulin ($n = 39$); and (6) three or more daily injections of insulin ($n = 15$).

Empirical testing for psychometric properties was conducted among two samples of participants whose diabetes was difficult to control ($n = 89$ and $n = 142$) in the initial and hypothesis testing phases, respectively. Because these participants required intensive inpatient diabetes management, the findings must be interpreted in that light. Another diabetes characteristic, degree of metabolic control at the time participants were administered the IMDSES, indicates that half of the sample could be defined as having uncontrolled diabetes.

Glycosylated hemoglobin (GH) is a minor hemoglobin fraction that is interpreted as a "marker" for the average blood glucose level during the past few months. GH develops slowly throughout the 120-day life span of the red blood cells. The measurement of GH represents the average amount of GH in the red cells, and GH levels have demonstrated reliability as a measure of overall blood glucose levels over a 2– to 3-month period (Grossman et al., 1987). High GH levels are associated with high blood glucose levels. All GH levels were measured by use of the Glytrac system, distributed by Corning Medical, Corning Glass Works. The nondiabetic range is 5.4% to 7.4%.

Patients who use insulin and are cared for at the setting used for this study are encouraged to maintain their GH below 11%. Of the participants who had a recent report of GH in their medical record (n = 127), half were in a state of metabolic control that required correction. Both the median and the mean GH were 10.9 (SD = 2.36). The range of values was 6.5 to 18.9.

Descriptive Data: Subscales and Scale Total

Mean scores were used on the scales and IMDSES total. To compute the means for the subscales, if participants had answered all but two items on a subscale, their mean score for the other items was substituted for the missing value(s). Likewise, for the scale total, if participants had responded to 20 of the 28 items, their total mean score was substituted for the missing value(s) to compute the scale total mean for the sample. Otherwise, participants were not included in the descriptive data reported. Comparisons of the scale and subscale means between the outpatient and inpatient participants revealed that there were no differences between the scores (all t tests were small and statistically not significant).

RELIABILITY AND VALIDITY

Initial Empirical Testing: Internal Consistency

Cronbach's alpha for the scale total (.82) revealed that the IMDSES achieved a reliability estimate considered adequate for a new scale (Nunnally, 1978). The Diet subscale had the highest alpha coefficients across the samples. The General subscale for the inpatient sample had an alpha over .70, but it was only .68 for the combined sample. The Insulin subscale, consisting of items dealing with monitoring, insulin administration and dose adjustment, and prevention, detection, and treatment of high and low blood sugars, had the lowest alpha coefficients. This can be explained by the range and complexity of behaviors that constitute the subscale. At this point, all items were considered essential to maintain content validity and were retained.

Retest Stability

Self-efficacy is a dynamic concept that theoretically can be altered by interventions that change any of its antecedents. Therefore, a homogeneous and stable group of participants was hypothesized to provide a moderate coefficient of stability, evidence for instrument stability. A convenience sample of 130 outpatients was identified through a medical records review. Potential participants were mailed a packet of information consisting of a letter of introduction and instructions, informed consents, and survey materials. Thirty-eight participants (29%) chose to participate, and 27 of those (71%) provided data for the examination of retest stability. Two weeks after participants returned the initial packet, a second was mailed; there was a mean duration of 22 days between test and retest. Given a dynamic concept but a stable sample, the Pearson correlation (r = .58, p < .002) was considered evidence of instrument stability. Paired t tests, $t(24)$ = .59, p < .56, revealed that the scale means and variance were unchanged from the test (M = 4.95) to the retest (M = 5.007), providing additional confirmation of instrument stability.

Convergent Validity

Two measures, the Insulin Management Diabetes Self Care Scale (IMD-SCS) and GH, provided evidence to support the convergent validity of the IMDSES. During the initial revision and testing of the IMDSES, an item-for-item self-report measure, the IMDSCS, was developed. If the self-efficacy item was "I can follow my diet plan when I go to parties," the corollary self-care item in the IMDSCS was "I followed my diet plan when I went to parties." The 28-item IMDSCS (the Care scale) was administered to all participants, before they responded to the IMDSES (the Efficacy scale), as part of the pilot test for all of the measures and procedures that would then be used in a prospective study.

The IMDSCS had been examined along with the IMDSES during the two phases of empirical testing, and the 28-item scale was also considered to have an adequate reliability estimate for a new scale. Cronbach's alpha was .96, N = 48. More of the 127 participants provided data for computing the reliability estimates for the three subscales, and those alpha coefficients were (1) six General items (.91, n = 120), (2) seven Diet items (.93, n = 110), and (3) 11 Insulin items (.88, n = 92). Retest stability of the IMDSCS indicated that it was a stable measure (r = .859, n = 27, p = .000) and that the means were unchanged from the test (M = 4.84) to the retest (M = 4.86) 22 days later, $t(26)$ = .32, p = .751.

There is not a direct correspondence between GH levels and self-care behaviors, especially in individuals who have type I diabetes, with fluctuating extremes of high and low blood glucose levels or a regimen in need of adjustment in order to promote good metabolic control. For participants who had been following a regimen that was correct for meeting their metabolic needs, if they were also correct in making their assessment of previous diabetes behaviors and if the IMDSCS accurately captured that information, then reported self-care behaviors should be negatively associated with the biochemical marker of "good control." However, as stated by Rapley and Furin (1999), adherence with all aspects of a recommended self-care regimen will not necessarily result in good metabolic control for the person with type 1 diabetes.

Therefore, the IMDSCS, IMDSES, GH, and two additional variables that had been a part of the sociodemographic scale—perception of previous metabolic control (CDB) and expectation for future metabolic control (CDA)—as well as GH levels, were examined in a correlation matrix. The CDB is scored so that high scores mean uncontrolled diabetes, and CDA is scored so that high scores mean an expectation of well-controlled diabetes in the future.

Pearson correlations revealed the following associations: (1) IMDSES/ IMDSCS: $r = +.376$, $n = 122$, $p = 000$; (2) IMDSCS/GH: $r = -.1738$, $n = 113$, $p = .033$; (3) GH/CDB: $r = +.2708$, $n = 116$, $p = .002$; (4) CDB/ IMDSCS: $r = -.4388$, $n = 123$, $p = .000$; and (5) CDA/IMDSES: $r = +.1687$, $n = 121$, $p = .032$. The IMDSCS and IMDSES were positively correlated as expected, because past behavior may be cognitively interpreted as enactive attainment, an antecedent of efficacy. GH and IMDSCS had a small negative association, meaning that the higher the score on the IMDSCS, the lower or "better" the GH. Thus, the association between GH (the biochemical marker of diabetes control) and IMDSCS (reported self-care), and the association between IMDSCS (interpreted in this case as the primary antecedent of self-efficacy, enactive attainment) and the IMDSES, support the construct validity of the self-efficacy scale. CDB (perception of control before) was positively associated with GH, and both were negatively related to the IMDSCS. CDA (expectation for a positive outcome) had a weak positive correlation with the IMDSES. These associations, even though small, collectively provide evidence to support construct validity of the IMDSES.

Hypothesis Testing Phase: Internal Consistency

Item analysis revealed that two items (numbers 19 and 20) were answered positively by almost all participants and were thus removed from further analyses. Cronbach's alpha for the scale total for the IMDSES was .86, above the standard of .80 expected for a mature scale (Nunnally & Bernstein, 1994). Alpha coefficients for the subscales were .67 for the General subscale, .78 for the Diet subscale, and .77 for the Insulin subscale.

Predictive Validity

On the day of discharge from the inpatient diabetes unit, participants ($N = 167$) completed the IMDSES and were mailed the IMDSCS (Hurley, 1990a) 2 weeks after discharge. One hundred and forty-two participants returned the IMDSCS within 2 weeks and are included in the analysis. The IMDSCS is an exact corollary of the IMDSES, item for item, but the stem is changed from "I can" to "I did" and is scored similarly. The efficacy assertion prior to discharge predicted diabetes self-care behaviors within a month of discharge. The 26-item IMDSCS scale total mean was 4.81 ($SD = .7$), and the Pearson correlation between scale total means was .58, accounting for 37% of the variance in IMDSCS scores (Hurley & Shea, 1992).

Analysis of the microanalytic match between the specific behavior of the efficacy assertion (IMDSES subscales) and subsequent behavior (IMD-SCS subscales) revealed positive associations. Pearson correlations were General Management $r = .40$, $p < .001$, Diet $r = .37$, $p < .001$, and Insulin $r = .67$, $p < .001$ (Hurley & Shea, 1992).

CONCLUSIONS AND RECOMMENDATIONS

The IMDSES is considered to have adequate psychometric properties of reliability by internal consistency evaluations conducted in three samples and stability. The methods of scale development built in content validity, which was demonstrated empirically. Adequate levels of both construct and predictive validity were obtained.

During the initial testing, all items were considered essential to maintain content validity and were retained. During hypothesis testing, two items were deleted. The IMDSES instructions call for administrating that scale with all 28 items and analyzing 26. Researchers may use their own judgment and use either the 26- or 28-item IMDSES. To compare future research findings with the hypothesis testing results, the 26-item scale should be used. To compare cross-cultural differences among English and Hispanic persons, the 28-item version, which has been translated into Spanish (Bernal et al., 2000), should be used.

Self-efficacy is a dynamic concept that has well-identified antecedents that may be enhanced or decreased by nursing interventions. When actions specific for managing diabetes regimens change individuals' interpretations of self-efficacy antecedents in a positive direction, the relative level of self-efficacy should increase. This result should lead to individuals' engaging in increased effort and persistence in carrying out those behaviors associated with good metabolic control of diabetes. Nurses could also use the IMDSES in clinical practice to aid in determining if there has been a positive change in patients' insulin management self-efficacy as a result of the implementation of teaching interventions.

REFERENCES

Bandura, A. (1977). Self-efficacy: Toward a unifying theory of behavior change. *Psychological Review, 84,* 191–215.

Bandura, A. (1982). Self-efficacy mechanism in human agency. *American Psychologist, 37*(2), 122–147.

Bandura, A. (1986). *Social foundations of thought and action: A social cognitive theory.* Englewood Cliffs, NJ: Prentice-Hall.

Bandura, A., & Adams, N. E. (1977). Analysis of self-efficacy theory of behavior change. *Cognitive Therapy and Research, 1,* 287–310.

Bandura, A., Adams, N., & Beyer, J. (1977). Cognitive processes mediating behavioral change. *Journal of Personality and Social Psychology, 35,* 125–139.

Bandura, A., Adams, N. E., Hardy, A. B., & Howells, G. N. (1980). Tests of the generality of self-efficacy theory. *Cognitive Therapy and Research, 4,* 39–66.

Bandura, A., Reese, L., & Adams, N. (1982). Microanalysis of action and fear arousal as a function of differential levels of perceived self-efficacy. *Journal of Personality and Social Psychology, 43,* 5–21.

Bernal, H., Woolley, S., Schensul, J. J., & Dickinson, J. K. (2000). Correlates of self-efficacy in diabetes self-care among Hispanic adults with diabetes. *Diabetes Educator, 26,* 673–680.

Coelho, R. J. (1984). Self-efficacy and cessation of smoking. *Psychological Reports, 54,* 309–310.

Colletti, G., Supnick, J. A., & Payne, T. J. (1985). The smoking self-efficacy questionnaire (SSEQ): Preliminary scale development and validation. *Behavioral Assessment, 7,* 249–260.

Condiotte, N. M., & Lichtenstein, E. (1981). Self-efficacy and relapse in smoking cessation programs. *Journal of Consulting and Clinical Psychology, 49,* 648–658.

Corbett, C. F. (1999). Research-based practice implications for patients with diabetes. Part 2: Diabetes self-efficacy. *Home Healthcare Nurse, 17,* 587–596.

Crabtree, M. K. (1986). *Self-efficacy and social support as predictors of diabetic self-care.* Unpublished doctoral dissertation, University of California, San Francisco.

Day, J. L. (2000). Diabetic patient education: Determinants of success. *Diabetes Metabolism and Research Review, 16*(Suppl. 1), S70–S74.

DiClemente, C. C. (1981). Self-efficacy and smoking cessation maintenance: A preliminary report. *Cognitive Therapy and Research, 5,* 175–187.

DiClemente, C., Prochaska, J. O., & Gibertini, M. (1985). Self-efficacy and the stages of self-change of smoking. *Cognitive Therapy and Research, 9,* 181–200.

Engel, S. S., Crandall, J., Basch, C. E., Zybert, P., & Wylie-Rosett J. (1997). Computer-assisted diabetes nutrition education increases knowledge and self-efficacy of medical students. *Diabetes Educator, 23,* 545–549.

Glasgow, R. E., and Osteen, V. L. (1992). Evaluating diabetes education: Are we measuring the most important outcomes? *Diabetes Care, 5,* 1423–1432.

Grossman, H. Y., Brink, S., & Hauser, S. (1987). Self-efficacy in adolescent girls and boys with insulin-dependent diabetes mellitus. *Diabetes Care, 10,* 324–329.

Hurley, A. C. (1990a). The health belief model: Evaluation of a diabetes scale. *Diabetes Educator, 16*(1), 44–48.

Hurley, A. C. (1990b). Measuring self-care ability in patients with diabetes: The Insulin Management Diabetes Self-Efficacy Scale. In C. Waltz & O. Strickland (Eds.), *Measurement of nursing outcomes: Measuring client self-care and coping skills* (pp. 28–44). New York: Springer Publishing Co.

Hurley, A. C., & Shea, C. A. (1992). Self-efficacy: Strategy for enhancing diabetes self-care. *Diabetes Educator, 18,* 146–150.

Johnson, J. A. (1996). Self-efficacy theory as a framework for community pharmacy-based diabetes education programs. *Diabetes Educator, 22,* 237–241.

Joslin Diabetes Center. (1986). *Diabetes teaching guide* (rev. ed.). Boston: Author.

Kneckt, M. C., Syrjala, A. M., Laukkanen, P., Knuuttila, M. L. (1999). Self-efficacy as a common variable in oral health behavior and diabetes adherence. *European Journal of Oral Science, 107*(2), 89–96.

Littlefield, C. H., Craven, J. L., Rodin, G. M., Daneman, D., Murray, M. A., & Rydall, A. C. (1992). Relationship of self-efficacy and bringing to adherence to diabetes regimen among adolescents. *Diabetes Care, 15*(1), 90–94.

Lorenz, R., Gregory, R. P., & Davis, D. L. (2000). Utility of a brief self-efficacy scale in clinical training program evaluation. *Evaluation in the Health Professions, 23,* 182–193. Lynn, M. (1986). Determination and quantification of content validity. *Nursing Research, 35,* 382–385.

McIntyre, K. O., Lichtenstein, E., & Mermelstein, R. J. (1983). Self-efficacy and relapse in smoking cessation: A replication and extension. *Journal of Consulting and Clinical Psychology, 51,* 632–633.

Nunnally, J. C. (1978). *Psychometric theory.* New York: McGraw-Hill.

Nunnally, J. C., & Bernstein, I. H. (1994). *Psychometric theory* (3rd ed.). New York: McGraw-Hill.

O'Leary, A. (1985). Self-efficacy and health. *Behavior Research and Therapy, 23,* 437–451.

Prochaska, J. O., Crimi, P., Lapsanski, D., Martel, L., & Reid, P. (1982). Self change processes, self-efficacy, and self concept in relapse and maintenance of cessation of smoking. *Psychological Reports, 51,* 983–990.

Senecal, C., Nouwen, A., & White, D. (2000). Motivation and dietary self-care in adults with diabetes: Are self-efficacy and autonomous self-regulation complementary or competing constructs? *Health Psychology, 19*(5), 452–457.

Skelly, A. H., Marshall, J. R., Haughey, B. P., Davis, P. J., & Dunford, R. G. (1995). Self-efficacy and confidence in outcomes as determinants of self-care practices in inner-city, African-American women with non-insulin-dependent diabetes. *Diabetes Educator, 21,* 38–46.

Telch, M. J., Bandura, A., Vinciguerra, P., Agras, A., & Stout, A. L. (1982). Social demand for consistency and congruence between self-efficacy and performance. *Behavior Therapy, 13,* 694–701.

APPENDIX: DIABETES MANAGEMENT BELIEFS SURVEY

The following statements describe what some people believe about their ability to take care of their diabetes. Please take the next few minutes to tell me what you believe about your ability to manage your diabetes. After reading each statement, circle the number that best expresses your beliefs. There are twenty-eight (28) statements, please answer each one. There are no right or wrong answers.

In this section, please indicate whether you agree or disagree with each of the items.

Circle 1 if you strongly agree with the statement.
        2 if you moderately agree with the statement.
        3 if you slightly agree with the statement.
        4 if you slightly disagree with the statement.
        5 if you moderately disagree with the statement.
        6 if you strongly disagree with the statement.
    NA if the statement does not apply to you.

	Strongly Agree	Moderately Agree	Slightly Agree	Slightly Disagree	Moderately Disagree	Strongly Disagree	Not Applicable
Example: I can test my urine for sugar before meals when I am away from home.							
Answer: If you are confident in your ability to test your urine before meals when you eat out, you should circle 1 because that statement best expresses your belief. If you do not test urine, you should circle NA (not applicable).	1	2	3	4	5	6	NA
1. I can carry out practically all of the self-care activities in my daily diabetes routine.	1	2	3	4	5	6	NA
2. I am confident in my ability to manage my diabetes.	1	2	3	4	5	6	NA
3. I feel unsure about having to use what I know about diabetes self-treatment every day.	1	2	3	4	5	6	NA
4. I don't think I can follow my diabetes routines every single day.	1	2	3	4	5	6	NA
5. I can eat my meals at the same time every day.	1	2	3	4	5	6	NA
6. I can stay on my diabetic diet when I eat in familiar places away from home (such as at a friend's house).	1	2	3	4	5	6	NA

	Strongly Agree	Moderately Agree	Slightly Agree	Slightly Disagree	Moderately Disagree	Strongly Disagree	Not Applicable
7. I can stay on my diabetic diet when I eat in unfamiliar places.	1	2	3	4	5	6	NA
8. I'm not sure I'll be able to stay on my diabetic diet when the people around me don't know that I have diabetes.	1	2	3	4	5	6	NA
9. I'm not sure I'll be able to follow my diabetic diet every day.	1	2	3	4	5	6	NA
10. I can correctly exchange one food for another in the same food group.	1	2	3	4	5	6	NA
11. When I go to parties, I can follow my diet plan.	1	2	3	4	5	6	NA
12. I can exercise several times a week.	1	2	3	4	5	6	NA
13. I can't exercise unless I feel like exercising.	1	2	3	4	5	6	NA
14. I can figure out when to call my doctor about problems with my feet.	1	2	3	4	5	6	NA
15. I can routinely apply the recommended lotion to my feet.	1	2	3	4	5	6	NA
16. I cannot test my blood or urine when I am away from home.	1	2	3	4	5	6	NA
17. I can recognize when my blood sugar is too high.	1	2	3	4	5	6	NA
18. When I feel sick, I can test my blood or urine more than I routinely do.	1	2	3	4	5	6	NA
19. I can take my insulin using the recommended procedure.	1	2	3	4	5	6	NA
20. I may have difficulty taking my insulin when away from home.	1	2	3	4	5	6	NA
21. I can adjust my insulin dose based on the results of my urine or blood tests.	1	2	3	4	5	6	NA
22. I'm not sure I can figure out what to do about my insulin dose when changes occur in my usual routine.	1	2	3	4	5	6	NA
23. I can do what was recommended to prevent low blood sugar reactions when I exercise.	1	2	3	4	5	6	NA
24. I can figure out what self-treatment to administer when my blood sugar gets higher than it should be.	1	2	3	4	5	6	NA
25. I'm not sure I can recognize when my blood sugar is low.	1	2	3	4	5	6	NA

	Strongly Agree	Moderately Agree	Slightly Agree	Slightly Disagree	Moderately Disagree	Strongly Disagree	Not Applicable
26. I'm not sure I can adjust my diabetes self-treatments if I get a cold or the flu.	1	2	3	4	5	6	NA
27. I can fit my diabetes self-treatment routine into my usual life style.	1	2	3	4	5	6	NA
28. I think I'll be able to follow my diabetes plan even when my daily routine changes.	1	2	3	4	5	6	NA

Please add any comments you wish about confidence in your ability to self manage diabetes.

Administration and Scoring:

The IMDSES is a paper and pencil test including 28 items and Likert responses ranging from 1 (*strongly agree*) to 6 (*strongly disagree*). A "not applicable" category is provided and is coded as missing data for computing reliability estimates. Eighteen positively worded items (1, 2, 5, 6, 7, 10, 11, 12, 14, 15, 17, 18, 19, 21, 23, 24, 27, 28) are reverse-scored, resulting in higher scores for individuals with a higher level of self-efficacy. Two of the items (19 and 20) were removed from the original scale analysis because they were answered positively by all test participants. You may use either the 26 or 28 items in scoring; however, for comparison with findings reported in the preceding work, only the 26 items should be used.

Mean scores of item groups, subscales, and the total IMDSES range from 1 (lowest) to 6 (highest). The total IMDSES score ranges from 26 to 156. Subscale totals (General: 1 to 4, plus 27 and 28) (Diet: 5 to 11) (Insulin: 16 to 26) may also be used. Note that the Insulin subscale includes items 19 and 20, which were deleted from the scoring. Two items about foot care (12 and 13), and two items about exercise (14 and 15) were considered too few to comprise subscales.

Subscale Mean Scores: If participants have answered all but two items of a subscale, the mean of the completed items is substituted for the missing value(s). The mean of the subscale is then calculated using the completed and substituted values.

IMDSES Mean Score: If participants have responded to 20 of the 28 scale items, the mean of the completed items is substituted for the missing items, and the mean for the total scale is calculated using the completed and substituted values. In the preceding published study, data were not included in the analysis if participants had not completed 20 of the 28 items.

PART II
Coping

6

The Jalowiec Coping Scale

Anne Jalowiec

This chapter discusses the Jalowiec Coping Scale, a measure of coping behavior across a wide range of stressful situations.

PURPOSE

This chapter will summarize how the Jalowiec Coping Scale (JCS) has been used by researchers and clinicians, will briefly describe the original version of the JCS, will discuss how the JCS was revised and why, and will summarize some of the psychometric support for the revised instrument.

The Jalowiec Coping Scale was designed to measure coping behavior across a wide range of stressful situations. The JCS has been used to assess coping with many kinds of physical, emotional, and social stressors, such as stressors associated with a wide variety of illnesses, major life stressors (e.g., loss of a loved one), family-related stressors, work-related stressors, and even stressors due to natural disasters (e.g., volcanic eruptions and hurricanes).

The instrument has been used in numerous studies nationwide and also internationally (including in Iceland, China, Turkey, Israel, Iran, India, and Thailand), and thus far the instrument has been translated into more than 20 languages. A variety of disciplines has employed the JCS for both research and clinical projects and sometimes also for intervention evaluation studies.

The JCS is appropriate for adults of all ages (including adolescents and elderly) and for both clinical and well populations. In terms of clinical populations, the instrument has been used with patients having many different kinds of illnesses (from relatively minor to life-threatening), both physical and emotional; also, much research has been done with this tool in family members of patients. In addition, the JCS has been used to assess how patients cope with the stress of invasive diagnostic procedures (e.g., breast biopsy).

CONCEPTUAL BASIS

Lazarus and Folkman (1984) pointed out that a taxonomy of coping styles needed to be developed to systematize research efforts. Such a taxonomy would provide a framework for generating researchable questions to investigate relationships between particular types of coping behavior and positive versus negative outcomes in health, functional status (physical, emotional, social), and quality of life. A taxonomy cannot be developed without examining conceptualizations of coping behavior in the literature. Some classification schemes have applied descriptive labels to the coping behavior (e.g., intrapsychic), whereas other labels were goal-oriented (e.g., maintain self-esteem) or evaluative (e.g., mature vs. immature). Although a few themes did recur (e.g., cognitive vs. behavioral, active vs. passive), for the most part, there seemed to be little consensus on the salient dimensions of coping behavior that should be measured.

Despite this confusion over the appropriate classification of coping strategies, the most popular conceptualization of coping behavior at the time of development of the JCS was the bidimensional schemata of problem-focused versus emotion-focused coping methods developed by Lazarus (Lazarus, 1966; Lazarus & Launier, 1978). This conceptual foundation was the basis for the original JCS.

JCS

I began to develop the first version of the Jalowiec Coping Scale in 1977 for my thesis research on stress and coping in hypertensive patients and emergency room patients (Jalowiec & Powers, 1981). I decided to develop the scale because instrumentation then available to assess coping behavior either was of the interview type or covered only a limited range of coping strategies or else was applicable to only a select population. The new instrument was meant to be broadly based and generic enough to cover a wide range of stressor situations.

The original JCS had 40 items that measured how often a person used each of the coping strategies listed. The items were obtained from a review of the stress and coping literature and included both behavioral and cognitive coping strategies. Based on Lazarus's writings, the items were classified by a panel of 20 nursing faculty and graduate students into 15 "problem-oriented" coping strategies (which focused on problem resolution) and 25 "affective-oriented" strategies (which were aimed at mitigation of distress). The use of each coping method was rated on a Likert-type scale from 1 (*never used*) to 5 (*always used*). A graded response format was employed for the JCS because it would yield more discriminating power than a dichotomous yes/no coping checklist (as were some coping tools of the time), and thus would better maximize the magnitude of the relationships between coping behavior and other variables.

It should be noted that a preliminary exploratory factor analysis with a small sample of 141 subjects did not support the hypothesized two-factor structure of the original JCS and yielded a four-factor solution instead (Jalowiec, Murphy, & Powers, 1984). Subsequently, confirmatory factor analysis from my 1985 dissertation on 1,400 subjects (published in the first edition of this measurement book: Jalowiec, 1988) later suggested a trichotomous classification of the coping items on the original JCS, labeled as confrontive, emotive, and palliative coping styles. This classification has since been used by some investigators.

The JCS was revised in 1987 (this is the version currently in use), with the following changes made: (1) The stressor of interest for the coping assessment was added, (2) more coping strategies were added, (3) the response format was changed, (4) a coping effectiveness component was added, and (5) the conceptualization of coping was expanded. Each change will be described below, along with the rationale for the change.

Targeted Stressor

Unlike the original JCS, the revised JCS includes a place on the cover page for the researcher or clinician to type in or write in the targeted stressor for the coping assessment. In addition, a time frame may be added to the stressor, for example, "I am interested in how you have coped with the stress of having had a heart transplant, in the last 3 months since you have come home from the hospital." Listing the targeted stressor will help the subject to stay focused on the appropriate stressor of interest while completing the JCS, so that the measurement process is more accurate.

More Coping Strategies

Based on my own empirical work, I felt that some important coping strategies were missing from the original JCS, which were needed to tap an even wider domain of coping behavior, in order to more accurately capture the richness and diversity of a person's coping repertoire. Therefore, I conducted a comprehensive review of the stress and coping literature to identify additional items for the instrument, as will be described.

Each time a coping strategy was mentioned in the literature, it was written on an index card, in addition to the number of times a particular coping method was cited. The literature review was conducted until the point of saturation, that is, until no new coping strategies were found that sounded different from the ones already recorded on the index cards. Once the literature review was completed, I then collated the index cards into piles of coping strategies that seemed alike. Coping methods that did not sound like any of the ones already on the original JCS were then added to the scale from these piles of cards. However, items that were scarcely mentioned in the literature (e.g., sexual activity as a way of coping) were not used because of concern for the instrument becoming too unwieldy for use in clinical settings.

In addition, based on my previous empirical and statistical work, some of the items from the original scale were eliminated, and some that seemed similar to another item on the JCS were combined with that item. Also, some of the original items were reworded to either simplify the wording to enhance understanding or to clarify the intent of the item so as to increase the precision of the measurement process. All of these steps resulted in the expansion of the JCS from 40 items on the original version to 60 items on the revised version. In addition, a section was now provided at the end of the instrument for subjects to write in (and rate) other coping strategies that they have used that are not already listed on the JCS.

Response Format

During subsequent years of use of the original JCS, several problems became apparent that prompted the need for the response format to be changed. First, my research using the JCS after my thesis work and then review of my dissertation data ($n = 1,400$) indicated that subjects were not making full use of the entire range of the possible responses on the 5-point rating scale on the original JCS. Therefore, they probably were not able to differentiate in their own minds the finer discrimination in the degree of use of the coping methods that the 5-point scale was attempting to measure.

My empirical work suggested that persons seem more comfortable with a simpler trichotomous measurement gradation corresponding to *a little, a medium amount,* and *a lot.* Therefore, on the 1987 revised JCS, the response format was changed to three levels (but using slightly different labels for the three gradations), plus a response option to indicate non-use of a coping strategy, thereby resulting in a 4-point rating scale. So the JCS response choices were now *never used* (0), *seldom used* (1), *sometimes used* (2), and *often used* (3).

Even though my first version of the JCS did allow for a nonuse option, the lower end of the rating scale started with 1 instead of 0. It became apparent that this type of rating system artificially inflated scores because if, for example, a person did not use any of the 40 coping strategies on the JCS, then he or she would still receive a total score of 40, not a score of 0 to indicate no use of any of the strategies. Thus, the score would be artificially inflated and not useful in conceptually interpreting the meaning of the results. Therefore, the rating scheme for the revised JCS was changed to start with 0 to indicate nonuse of a coping strategy.

In addition, at the upper end of the rating scale, the descriptive anchor was changed from the original *always used* to *often used*, because logically a person would not be able to use any particular coping method "all of the time" due to different constraining conditions existing in different situations.

Coping Effectiveness

In addition to rating the degree of use of each coping method, the JCS was revised to allow evaluation of the effectiveness of each coping strategy, as perceived by the subject. This component was missing from other instruments of that time, and I felt that coping assessments would benefit from incorporating this evaluative dimension. One reason was that a person may not necessarily use to a greater degree those strategies that have been found to be most effective in the past, thereby leading to an incongruence between use and effectiveness. Moreover, if a person feels that a particular coping method was effective in a specific situation, then the person would probably not continue to search for other ways of coping with that stressor, and may feel more at ease about his or her confidence in handling the situation, which should reduce stress and enhance self-esteem.

However, some researchers may feel that perceived effectiveness is too subjective, and that some objective measure of effectiveness be used instead. So objective measures of coping effectiveness can be added to the JCS assessment, such as specific instruments to evaluate the level of stress or anxiety or well-being afterwards, or any other number of possible psychological outcomes of adaptive coping behavior. Clinical outcomes of coping effectiveness can also be examined, for example, by measuring the blood sugar of a patient with diabetes to determine if patients who cope with the demands of their illness in a constructive manner demonstrate better control of their blood sugar.

Therefore, the 1987 revised JCS asks the subject to also rate how helpful each coping strategy (that was used) has been in coping with the stressor listed on the cover page of the scale. The response format for effectiveness is also on a 4-point scale: *not helpful in reducing stress* (0), *slightly helpful* (1), *fairly helpful* (2), and *very helpful* (3).

Multidimensional Coping

Because the exploratory and confirmatory factor analyses cited earlier indicated that a dichotomous classification of the coping strategies on the original JCS was too simplistic a conceptualization, a multidimensional conceptual approach to coping behavior was needed. Moreover, because 20 new items had been added to the revised scale, this also enlarged the domain of coping being measured and further emphasized the importance of examining a multidimensional classification of the coping items, rather than the bidimensional schemata based on the model by Lazarus.

Therefore, when the JCS was revised, I used sequential thematic clustering to rationally derive related clusters of similar coping strategies to generate a multidimensional model of coping behavior. This was done by first examining the list of the 60 coping strategies to identify all items that seemed to relate thematically to one type of coping behavior, for example, optimistic coping strategies. These items were removed from the list and grouped separately under the optimistic label.

The list of remaining items was again examined to identify coping strategies that pertained to a second type of coping behavior, for example, evasive coping. These items were also removed from the list and grouped separately under the evasive label. This procedure of thematic clustering was repeated sequentially until no coping items remained on the list.

This iterative process resulted in a multidimensional model of eight coping styles identified as those underlying the coping domains being measured by the revised JCS. (It should be noted that there was no a priori decision to derive eight subscales for the revised instrument.) Based on their thematic content, these coping styles were named as follows: confrontive, evasive, optimistic, fatalistic, emotive, palliative, supportant, and self-reliant. See Table 6.1 for a description and an example of each of these coping styles.

A point needs to be made about confrontive coping. The JCS confrontive coping style pertains to constructive problem-solving strategies that focus on confronting and facing up to the problem, rather than avoiding

TABLE 6.1 Coping Styles on Jalowiec Coping Scale

Coping style	Items	Description	Coping example
Confrontive	10	Face up to the problem	Figure out ways to handle problem
Evasive	13	Avoid the problem	Try to get away from the problem
Optimistic	9	Positive thinking	Try to think positively
Fatalistic	4	Pessimistic thinking	Expect the worst that could happen
Emotive	5	Release emotions	Get mad and let off steam
Palliative	7	Make yourself feel better	Take medications to reduce stress
Supportant	5	Use support systems	Discuss problem with family/ friends
Self-reliant	7	Depend on yourself	Feel you can handle things yourself

or evading it. Examples of confrontive coping strategies include trying to figure out different ways to handle the situation, trying to find out more about the problem so you can deal with it better, and trying to handle things one step at a time. In the past, I have encountered in the literature the use of the label *confrontative coping* as an alternative for *confrontive coping*. However, confrontative coping implies a conflict-ridden type of coping behavior (e.g., when you are involved in a confrontation with someone), not a constructive approach to handling the problem. Therefore, in my mind, these two labels should not be confused, nor should they be used interchangeably (although journal editors consistently try to change *confrontive* to *confrontative*). Thus, confrontive coping suggests a positive type of coping approach, whereas confrontative coping focuses on negative coping behavior.

ADMINISTRATION AND SCORING

To score the instrument, the ratings for the individual items are summed separately for each coping style. Two main types of scores can be derived from the 1987 revised JCS: use and effectiveness. These scores can be obtained for each of the eight coping styles and also for the overall scale if desired (i.e., overall use and overall effectiveness). Scores for each of the eight coping styles can be expressed either as raw scores or as adjusted scores.

Individualized Adjusted Scores

To calculate individualized adjusted scores, the raw use score and the raw effectiveness score for a coping style are each divided by the number of coping methods actually used by that subject for that particular coping style. This provides an idiosyncratic adjustment for the person's use and effectiveness of each coping style, and is therefore a more accurate assessment for comparative purposes, instead of the usual way of dividing by the number of items on the subscale. This type of individualized score adjusts for two conditions: (1) that there are different numbers of coping strategies on each subscale and (2) that a person typically does not use all of the coping methods for a particular coping style; some persons might use only a few of the strategies on a subscale.

When to Use Raw Scores and Adjusted Scores

Raw scores should be used only when comparing the same coping style between different groups. The maximum possible score for raw scores is

3 times the number of items on the subscale. Adjusted scores should be used when comparing different coping styles against each other for subjects within one group, or when comparing different coping styles between different groups. In addition, adjusted scores can be used any time raw scores are appropriate. The possible range of adjusted scores for the use and the effectiveness of each coping style (and also for overall use and overall effectiveness) is 0 to 3, the same range as for the ratings on the individual items.

Readability

Previously, I had used the Grammatik computer program to assess readability of the revised JCS and found a sixth-grade reading level. In addition, Gayleen Ienatsch (for her master's thesis, Texas Tech University; personal communication, 1994) used the Fry readability formula and found a third-grade reading level. More recently, as part of her National Institutes of Health (NIH) study, Dr. Kathleen Grady (Rush University, Chicago; personal communication, May 2000) contracted the Center for Literacy at the University of Illinois (Chicago) to assess the reading level of her study tools, including the revised JCS. The center performed six different readability analyses on the JCS, including the Flesch, the FOG Readability Test (Gunning, 1952) and the SMOG Readability Test (McLaughlin, 1969). Four of the six tests determined that the JCS has a fifth- to sixth-grade reading level, plus one test showed a second- to third-grade level. Therefore, the JCS can be readily understood by most persons.

Administration

The JCS can be easily self-administered in 10 to 15 minutes, because of its lower reading level. Instructions for completion are included on the cover page, along with an example for completing Part A on coping use and Part B on coping effectiveness.

RELIABILITY AND VALIDITY OF THE REVISED JCS

Some of the psychometric support for the revised JCS will be summarized below. Much of the data cited comes from my 10–year NIH study (#NR01693) on age and gender differences in multiple outcomes that affect the quality of life of heart transplant (HT) patients during the preoperative wait for a new heart and for 5 years after the surgery (coinvestigators on the NIH study: Dr. Kathleen Grady and Connie White-

Williams). Other psychometric data can be found in the many articles reporting on JCS studies; a bibliography is included in the JCS packet that is sent to persons requesting permission to use the instrument. In addition, a MEDLINE search (using the keywords "Jalowiec Coping Scale") can identify articles on JCS studies; however, keep in mind that MED-LINE will retrieve the article only if those specific keywords are in the abstract (i.e., many articles are missed in this narrow type of search).

Homogeneity Reliability

Table 6.2 lists recent Cronbach's alpha reliabilities on the revised JCS using data from my NIH HT study (n = 550 HT candidates) plus data from my coinvestigator's (Dr. Kathleen Grady) American Heart Association study

TABLE 6.2 Cronbach's Alpha Reliabilities for JCS Use and Effectiveness Scores Based on Studies on Heart Transplant Candidates by Jalowiec and by Grady

Scale	Jalowiec study (n = 550) Alpha	Grady study[1] (n = 81) Alpha
Total Use	.93	.87
Total EFF	.94	.90
Confrontive Use	.81	.84
Confrontive EFF	.79	.88
Evasive Use	.78	.84
Evasive EFF	.82	.87
Optimistic Use	.78	.86
Optimistic EFF	.71	.89
Fatalistic Use	.49	.86
Fatalistic EFF	.56	.89
Emotive Use	.63	.86
Emotive EFF	.63	.89
Palliative Use	.55	.84
Palliative EFF	.56	.88
Supportant Use	.63	.86
Supportant EFF	.56	.90
Self-reliant Use	.70	.83
Self-reliant EFF	.69	.87

[1]Grady et al. (2001).

EFF = effectiveness.

TABLE 6.3 Summary of Cronbach's Alpha Reliabilities for JCS Use and Effectiveness Scores Based on 25 Studies Conducted by Other Investigators from 1988 to 1994

Scale	Mean alpha	Highest alpha	Lowest alpha
Total Use	.85	.97	.57
Total EFF	.90	.97	.84
Confrontive Use	.80	.96	.68
Confrontive EFF	.81	.94	.61
Evasive Use	.72	.91	.12
Evasive EFF	.74	.89	.44
Optimistic Use	.70	.91	.45
Optimistic EFF	.75	.96	.55
Fatalistic Use	.53	.89	.18
Fatalistic EFF	.49	.89	.16
Emotive Use	.60	.89	.24
Emotive EFF	.58	.89	.11
Palliative Use	.47	.88	.03
Palliative EFF	.58	.90	.02
Supportant Use	.55	.89	.03
Supportant EFF	.61	.90	.08
Self-reliant Use	.61	.88	.02
Self-reliant EFF	.65	.88	.18

Note: List of investigators available upon request; sample sizes of studies ranged from 10 to 210.

EFF = effectiveness.

on HT candidates who are on left ventricular assist devices while awaiting a new heart ($n = 81$; Grady et al., 2001). In addition, Table 6.3 summarizes Cronbach's alpha reliabilities (unpublished data, 1998) on the revised JCS from 25 studies (conducted from 1988 to 1994) by other investigators who were kind enough to share their psychometric data with me ($n = 10$–210); a list of these researchers is available on request.

A review of these two tables shows that the alphas for the JCS total use score and for the total effectiveness score support homogeneity reliability of the overall scale. In examining subscale results on the table summarizing the 25 older studies (Table 6.3), it can be seen that the range of alphas (highest vs. lowest for each subscale) is very wide for most subscales. This is again noted on several subscales on the table comparing the two HT studies (Table 6.2). This wide range in alphas may be due to differences in the study populations and the stressor situations under examination, or it could be due to differences in scoring methods (early on, I had proposed several different methods for scoring the JCS).

Conclusions on homogeneity reliability of the JCS subscales are the following:

1. Three subscales showed strong homogeneity reliability: confrontive, evasive, and optimistic.
2. Three subscales are moderately strong: self-reliant, supportant, and emotive.
3. Two subscales have lower homogeneity: palliative and fatalistic.

It should be pointed out that the palliative subscale contains both desirable methods of stress reduction (e.g., exercising, relaxation) and undesirable methods (e.g., smoking, drinking), so this mixture may be lowering alpha. Note also that the fatalistic subscale has only four items, which could affect homogeneity reliability.

Stability Reliability

To assess stability reliability of the revised JCS, data from multiple preoperative and postoperative time periods from my NIH study on HT patients were examined. Correlations between time periods were run using retest intervals of 3, 6, 9, and 12 months (n for this data = 110–275). This yielded a total of 144 retest correlations (see Table 6.4 for use results and Table 6.5 for effectiveness results; unpublished data, 1995). Note that it was important to analyze preoperative time periods separately from postoperative time periods, because the stressors differ before and after HT surgery, which can affect the type of coping methods used.

Based on all the time periods examined, the JCS total use score showed a mean retest correlation of moderate magnitude at .61 (range = .56 to .69; Table 6.4). For the eight use subscales, the mean retest correlation was .55 (range = .37 to .70; Table 6.4). The three most stable coping styles in terms of use were emotive, evasive, and supportant coping behavior. The least stable over time was fatalistic coping.

For all the time periods examined, the JCS total effectiveness score also showed a mean retest correlation of moderate magnitude (although lower than the mean for the total use score) at .52 (range = .43 to .63; Table 6.5). For the eight effectiveness subscales, the mean retest correlation was .47 (range = .22 to .65; Table 6.5). The three most stable coping styles in terms of effectiveness were supportant, optimistic, and palliative coping. The least stable over time was again fatalistic coping.

Conclusions on stability reliability of the JCS subscales are the following:

1. All use subscales showed moderate stability reliability over 3 to 12-month retest intervals.

TABLE 6.4 Retest Correlations for JCS Total Use Score and for Use Subscales Using Jalowiec Heart Transplant Data

Scale	Retest interval				
	3 Months	6 Months	9 Months	12 Months	Mean
Total Use	.69	.66	.58	.60	.61
	.62	.56	.60	.56	
Confrontive Use	.63	.55	.47	.53	.54
	.59	.50	.53	.51	
Evasive Use	.67	.68	.61	.52	.59
	.62	.55	.56	.51	
Optimistic Use	.58	.54	.48.	.54	.55
	.62	.58	.55	.54	
Fatalistic Use	.52	.54	.52	.43	.46
	.47	.37	.37	.47	
Emotive Use	.60	.67	.60	.56	.60
	.57	.57	.65	.60	
Palliative Use	.65	.60	.63	.61	.56
	.51	.52	.50	.46	
Supportant Use	.65	.67	.63	.70	.58
	.49	.50	.52	.50	
Self-reliant Use	.58	.57	.52	.57	.54
	.57	.52	.52	.48	

Note: First row of each cell is preoperative data; second row is postoperative data. Preoperative sample sizes: 275 at 3 months, 182 at 6 months, 141 at 9 months, 110 at 12 months. Postoperative sample sizes: 208 at 3 months, 179 at 6 months, 167 at 9 months, 147 at 12 months.

2. All effectiveness subscales showed low to moderate stability reliability over time.
3. Use of the various coping styles showed greater stability than perceived effectiveness.
4. For some coping styles, there was a slight degradation in reliability for the longer retest intervals, especially for 12 months.

It should be pointed out that one reason that very high retest correlations were not demonstrated could be that the patients' coping behavior was gradually evolving over time as they were becoming more familiar with handling the demands of their illness and the HT surgery. In other words, the lack of very high retest stability (within each specific time period, preoperative vs. postoperative) may be more a function of the changing characteristics of the stressful situation, rather than due to less reliability of the instrument.

TABLE 6.5 Retest Correlations for JCS Total Effectiveness Score and for Effectiveness Subscales Using Jalowiec Heart Transplant Data

	Retest interval				
Scale	3 Months	6 Months	9 Months	12 Months	Mean
Total EFF	.63	.59	.49	.53	.52
	.58	.47	.46	.43	
Confrontive EFF	.57	.53	.46	.53	.51
	.56	.45	.47	.47	
Evasive EFF	.51	.58	.52	.44	.45
	.51	.38	.37	.31	
Optimistic EFF	.61	.59	.49	.56	.56
	.63	.59	.54	.49	
Fatalistic EFF	.43	.43	.40	.35	.34
	.38	.22.	24	.23	
Emotive EFF	.35	.40	.23	.38	.35
	.42	.41	.28	.31	
Palliative EFF	.58	.56	.62	.59	.52
	.52	.47	.43	.38	
Supportant EFF	.63	.61	.65	.65	.58
	.57	.49.	53	.53	
Self-reliant EFF	.54	.57	.35	.41	.48
	.54	.51	.49	.42	

Note: First row of each cell is preoperative data; second row is postoperative data. Preoperative sample sizes: 275 at 3 months, 182 at 6 months, 141 at 9 months, 110 at 12 months. Postoperative sample sizes: 208 at 3 months, 179 at 6 months, 167 at 9 months, 147 at 12 months.

EFF = effectiveness.

Content Validity

Support for the content validity of the JCS is based on (1) the large number of items used, (2) the broad literature review from which the coping items were generated, and (3) the inclusion of a wide range of behavioral and cognitive coping strategies.

Construct Validity

In 1987 after revising the JCS, I conducted an empirical construct validity study to try to confirm the dimensionality of the instrument as I had structured the subscales based on sequential thematic clustering. The purpose was to examine the extent to which a panel of 25 nurse researchers, who were familiar with the stress and coping literature (from the Stress and Coping section of the Midwest Nursing Research Society), agreed with my classification of the 60 JCS items into eight coping styles.

Panel members were given descriptions of each coping style and instructed to code each item as one of the eight styles. They were told to try to classify each item under only one coping style, but if they felt strongly that a coping strategy related to two styles, they could code it that way. Coding of the items was done independently by mail (not by group discussion), and the panel members were not aware of my classification of the items.

The highest agreement between the panel's coding and my own classification of the coping strategies was found on the supportant (94%) and confrontive items (86%). The lowest agreement was on the emotive (54%) and self-reliant items (66%). The mean percent of agreement for all eight subscales was 75%, and thus largely supported my rationally derived classification of the coping items using the process of sequential thematic clustering.

In further support of the construct validity of the JCS subscales, Ienatsch (master's thesis, Texas Tech University; personal communication, 1994) conducted an evaluation of how well the 60 items on the revised JCS related to the eight subscales, using a panel of three judges. In this case, the panel was aware of the composition of the subscales and was being asked if an item made sense on a particular subscale. Ienatsch obtained a validity index of .85 (out of a possible 1.00), thereby demonstrating strong support for the relevance of the JCS items to each of their respective subscales.

Concurrent and Predictive Validity

To document the concurrent and predictive validity of the revised JCS, examples from my NIH HT study are reported in Table 6.6 (*n* for this data = 150 to 550; unpublished data, 1995, 2001). Conclusions on concurrent and predictive validity of the JCS are the following:

1. Greater effectiveness of coping behavior was associated with better outcomes of many different kinds (e.g., higher quality of life, less stress, better social and emotional functioning, needing less help with illness-related tasks).
2. A greater use of less desirable coping behavior (evasive, fatalistic, emotive) was associated with poorer outcomes (e.g., less life satisfaction, more stress, more psychological symptoms, perception of a poor ability to cope with the illness).

Thus, the evidence provides strong support for the concurrent and predictive validity of the JCS.

TABLE 6.6 Examples of Concurrent and Predictive Validity Correlations for JCS Using Jalowiec Heart Transplant Data

Findings	r	p
Greater coping effectiveness correlated with:		
More satisfaction with life	.40	.000
Higher overall quality of life	.20	.000
Lower overall level of stress	−.31	.000
Fewer heart transplant stressors	−.29	.000
Better perceived ability to cope with the illness	.31	.000
Fewer psychological symptoms	−.29	.000
Better social functioning	−.26	.000
Better emotional functioning	−.28	.000
Better perception of health prognosis	.28	.000
Needing less help with illness-related tasks	.19	.025
Increased use of evasive coping correlated with:		
Less satisfaction with life	−.35	.000
Lower overall quality of life	−.23	.006
Higher overall level of stress	.48	.000
More psychological symptoms	.42	.000
Increased use of fatalistic coping correlated with:		
Less satisfaction with life	−.44	.000
Lower overall quality of life	−.26	.002
Higher overall level of stress	.43	.000
Worse perceived ability to cope with the illness	−.21	.001
More psychological symptoms	.29	.000
Poor perception of health status	−.24	.005
Increased use of emotive coping correlated with:		
Less satisfaction with life	−.45	.000
Lower overall quality of life	−.26	.002
Higher overall level of stress	.53	.000
Worse perceived ability to cope with the illness	−.33	.000
More psychological symptoms	.53	.000
Poor perception of health status	−.22	.008

Note: n = 150–550.

CONCLUSIONS AND RECOMMENDATIONS

In summary, the Jalowiec Coping Scale measures the degree of use and the perceived effectiveness of 60 cognitive and behavioral coping strategies, which are rated on 4-point Likert-type scales. The items are classified into eight coping styles: confrontive, evasive, optimistic, fatalistic, emotive, palliative, supportant, and self-reliant. Comparison of different coping styles is done with individualized adjusted scores. The JCS has been shown to have well-documented reliability and validity. Because the instrument has a fifth- to sixth-grade reading level, it is readily understood by most persons and therefore is easily self-administered. In conclusion, the JCS is a widely used questionnaire (both nationally and internationally) for examining relationships between the use and effectiveness of different kinds of coping behavior and a multitude of outcomes related to health, functioning, and quality of life. The instrument is applicable for diverse adult populations and for a broad range of stressors, and is therefore generic enough for most research and clinical uses. For permission to obtain, use or revise the Jalowiec Coping Scale, contact the author: Anne Jalowiec, RN, PhD, FAAN at her e-mail address: jalo@prodigy.net or ajalowiec@yahoo.com.

ACKNOWLEDGMENT

The study that provided the HT data for this report was funded by multiple sources for almost $3.5 million over a 10–year period. Therefore, I gratefully acknowledge these funding sources: 4 NIH grants (#NR01693, #NR01693/S, #2NR01693, #HL49336), Sandoz Pharmaceuticals Corporation, Earl Bane Estate, Sigma Theta Tau, American Association of Critical-Care Nurses, Loyola University of Chicago (School of Nursing, Dean's Research Fund, Nursing Research Committee, University Research Committee), and Loyola University Medical Center (Department of Thoracic and Cardiovascular Surgery, Department of Nursing Administration, Capital Budget Committee, Office of the Executive Vice President). Study principal investigator is Dr. Anne Jalowiec, now Professor Emerita, Loyola University of Chicago.

REFERENCES

Grady, K. L., Meyer, P., Mattea, A., White-Williams, C., Ormaza, S., Kaan, A., et al. (2001). Improvement in quality of life outcomes 2 weeks after left ventricular assist device implantation. *Journal of Heart and Lung Transplantation, 20,* 657–669.

Gunning, R. (1952). *The technique of clear writing.* New York: McGraw-Hill.

Jalowiec, A. (1988). Confirmatory factor analysis of the Jalowiec Coping Scale. In C. F. Waltz & O. L. Strickland (Eds.), *Measurement of nursing outcomes: Measuring client outcomes* (pp. 287–308). New York: Springer.

Jalowiec, A., Murphy, S. P., & Powers, M. J. (1984). Psychometric assessment of the Jalowiec Coping Scale. *Nursing Research, 33,* 157–161.

Jalowiec, A., & Powers, M. J. (1981). Stress and coping in hypertensive and emergency room patients. *Nursing Research, 30,* 10–15.

Lazarus, R. S. (1966). *Psychological stress and the coping process.* New York: McGraw-Hill.

Lazarus, R. S., & Folkman, S. (1984). *Stress, appraisal, and coping.* New York: Springer.

Lazarus, R. S., & Launier, R. (1978). Stress-related transactions between person and environment. In L. A. Pervin & M. Lewis (Eds.), *Perspectives in interactional psychology* (pp. 287–327). New York: Plenum.

McLaughlin, H. (1969). SMOG grading—A new readability formula. *Journal of Reading, 12,* 639–646.

7

The Coping Scale of the Chronicity Impact and Coping Instrument

Debra P. Hymovich

This chapter discusses the Coping Scale of the Chronicity Impact and Coping Instrument: Parent Questionnaire (CICI:PQ), a measure of the coping of parents with a chronically ill child.

PURPOSE

There are an increasing number of studies related to coping, chronic illness, and families. The majority of chronic illness studies deal with how adults with various illnesses cope with the problems they encounter. Studies related to how parents cope with a child's chronic illness are limited, often due to inadequate instruments to measure parental coping. Therefore, the purpose of this chapter is to describe the psychometric properties of the Coping scale of the Chronicity Impact and Coping Instrument: Parent Questionnaire (CICI:PQ) (Hymovich, 1983, 1984). The Coping scale of the CICI:PQ (Hymovich, 1981, 1983, 1984; Hymovich & Baker, 1985) was designed to measure how parents of chronically ill children cope with stressors related to their child's illness.

CONCEPTUAL BASIS OF THE COPING SCALE OF THE CHRONICITY IMPACT AND COPING INSTRUMENT: PARENT QUESTIONNAIRE

The CICLPQ Coping scale measures coping strategies used by parents of a chronically ill child. Although there are nearly as many definitions of coping as there are authors writing about it, there are several definitions that appear consistently in the chronic illness literature (Lazarus & Launier, 1978; Pearlin & Schooler, 1978; Weisman, 1984; Weisman & Worden, 1976–1977). Regardless of the specific definition, coping basically refers to a purposeful and intentional self-regulatory process that reduces or prevents responses that normally occur under stress (Burish & Bradley, 1983). Coping includes the behavioral responses of family members as well as the responses of the family as a unit in an attempt to manage a stressful situation. Within the family context, coping is the "ability to acquire and use the resources needed for family adaptation" (Patterson & McCubbin, 1983, p. 30). Coping may be conceptualized as a disposition (personality trait or style), a process (Averill & Opton, 1968), or an outcome (Stewart, 1980). Another way of conceptualizing coping is to consider it in relation to the concept of stress, either as an endocrinologic and physiologic process (Selye, 1976) or as an interactionist, cognitively oriented process (Folkman, Schaefer, & Lazarus, 1979). The CICI:PQ considers coping as an outcome behavior that occurs in response to stress.

The conceptual basis for the CICI:PQ was the evolving framework developed by Hymovich (1981, 1984). As the framework evolved, the coping instrument was modified to reflect the changes. The current framework states that coping strategies are parents' perceptions of what they do to manage problems faced in raising a chronically ill child. The conceptual definition of coping for the CICI:PQ is that of Weisman and Worden (1976–1977): "what one does about a perceived problem in order to bring about relief, reward, quiescence, or equilibrium" (p. 3). These strategies are either problem- or emotion-focused (Folkman & Lazarus, 1980), and may or may not be effective in resolving the problem (stressor) (Hymovich, 1987). Folkman and Lazarus (1980) differentiate between problem-focused and emotion-focused coping. Problem-focused coping refers to actions taken to remove or alleviate the source of stress, whereas emotion-focused coping refers to attempts to reduce the psychological distress, that is, to make the person feel better.

PROCEDURES FOR DEVELOPMENT

The CICI:PQ was developed in two phases. The first phase focused on developing the categories for the tool, including the list of coping strategies (behaviors). To elicit information about coping strategies, parents were asked to describe an incident that was stressful to them, what they did to manage the situation, and how effective their coping was in managing the situation. Content analysis of the tape-recorded interviews resulted in a coping category with seven subcategories of strategies: (1) seeking behaviors (to obtain information or resources), (2) utilizing behaviors (to make use of information and resources), (3) managing stressors (actions to manage the child's physical needs and parents' emotional responses), (4) modifying strategies (to alter conditions or situations affecting family functioning), (5) anticipatory planning, (6) educating others, and (7) helping/supporting others.

The second phase of the study consisted of developing the CICI:PQ and pilot-testing the instrument. The initial tool contained 213 coping items taken from the categories and subcategories. Three pilot tests were conducted with parents of chronically ill children. The sample sizes ranged from 29 to 44 parents. After a fourth revision, the 167-item tool was published (Hymovich, 1983) so that it could be used by other nurse-researchers.

DESCRIPTION

The CICI:PQ, developed in 1978, is a 167-item questionnaire with eight sections. The Coping scale consists of 39 items. Two of these sections include coping items. One set of items is related to coping strategies used by the person completing the instrument; the other set is related to that person's perceptions of spousal coping. A Likert-type format was used for the items comprising the Coping scale. The Coping scale consists of three subscales: COPECHLD (coping with problems and concerns related to the child's health), COPESPOU (coping when upset with spouse), and SPOUCOPE (parent's perception of how one's spouse copes when upset with the parent completing instrument). The COPECHLD and COPE-SPOU items can be combined to produce a SELFCOPE scale. Each subscale contains the same 13 coping strategies.

ADMINISTRATION AND SCORING

Parents are asked to indicate whether they used each coping strategy more, less, or about the same as under usual circumstances (see instrument in Appendix 1). Scoring of each scale consists of summing the subject's score to obtain a composite score. Items that are checked as being used (more, less, the same) can be given a score of 1, and the items not used can be given a score of 0. The total number of coping strategies is then summed to give the total number of strategies used for each subscale. Therefore, scores can range from 0 to 13 for the COPECHLD, COPESPOU, and SPOUCOPE subscales and 0 to 26 for the SELFCOPE scale. Higher scores indicate the use of more coping strategies. The means, standard deviations, and ranges for the CICI:PQ Coping scale for mothers and fathers can be found in Hymovich (1990).

RELIABILITY AND VALIDITY EVIDENCE

Sample

The sample for the psychometric analysis of the CICI:PQ consisted of 452 parents of children with a wide range of chronic illnesses from the United

States and Canada. The majority of the parents were White (86%), married (84%), and between 30 and 39 years of age (43%). Fifty-five percent of the sample had a 12th-grade education or lower, and 45% had at least some college education. Incomes ranged from under $10,000 per year (18%) to over $30,000 (35%). The remainder were evenly distributed between $11,000 and $30,000. Parents of children with cystic fibrosis represented approximately 40% of the sample; spina bifida, 19%; asthma, 16%; and other, 25%.

Reliability

Internal consistency reliability for the SELFCOPE and SPOUCOPE scales using Hoyt's coefficient was .80 for each. Internal consistency of the scales (Cope with Child, Cope with Spouse, Spouse cope, Self-Cope with Child and Spouse) for the sample of 452 parents was examined using Cronbach's alpha coefficient. Coefficients were determined separately for mothers and fathers and for mothers and fathers within four child disability categories. A coefficient alpha of .86 for mothers and .88 for fathers was obtained for the total Coping scale. Ranges of correlations between the subscales and the total scale score were .55 to .96 for mothers, and .41 to .95 for fathers. Internal consistency reliabilities of the scales for the three diagnostic groups ranged from .72 to .88 for the cystic fibrosis group, .68 to .84 for the spina bifida group, and .62 to .82 for the asthma group. When the diagnostic groups were combined, the only scale with an alpha coefficient below .70 was COPECHLD (.68).

Validity

Content Validity

A priori content validity of the CICI:PQ based on the identification categories and subcategories emerged from the parent interviews and a review of the literature. Content validity was also evident because the items in the instrument came from parents' statements of their coping behaviors during the interview phase of the tool's development. Posteriori content validity was assessed by submitting the CICI:PQ to a clinical psychologist, three nurses working with families of chronically ill children, and one nurse working with chronically ill adults. Each item of the CICI:PQ was screened to be certain that each category and subcategory was included in the instrument.

Construct Validity

Factor analysis was performed on the Coping scale data for 452 parents. Separate analyses were run for mothers ($n = 313$) and fathers ($n = 139$). The diagnostic categories were combined for the analyses.

Bartlett's test of sphericity indicated that there was sufficient correlation among the items to proceed with the analysis. Because not all parents in the sample were married and could not respond to the entire Coping scale, it was decided to look at each of the scales separately. The number of items in each of the three subscales analyzed was 13. The subscales were COPECHLD (cope with child), COPESPOU (cope with spouse), and SPOUCOPE (how spouse copes).

The principal-components method was used to determine the number of eigenvalues of 1.00 or greater as a cutoff for determining the number of potentially interpretable factors in the data, and was followed by a varimax (orthogonal) factor rotation. The initial varimax solution for mothers yielded four factors for the COPECHLD scale, five for the COPESPOU scale, and three for SPOUCOPE. For the fathers, the COPECHLD and COPESPOU sub-scales yielded five factors each, and the SPOUCOPE scale yielded three factors. These findings suggest that coping is a multidimensional concept, especially in relation to the affective domain.

The four-factor solution was the most meaningful conceptually. The factors were named avoidance behaviors, seeking emotional support, problem solving and exercise, and tension-reducing activities. The most consistent factors across the three subscales for mothers and fathers were avoidance behaviors and tension-reducing activities. These findings are consistent with those of Aldwin and colleagues (Aldwyn, Folkman, Schaefer, Coyne, & Lazarus, 1980), who used principal-components analysis with varimax rotation to empirically determine the coping strategies in Folkman and Lazarus's Ways of Coping Checklist. Of the seven factors, one problem-focused and six emotion-focused coping factors were derived. The items and factor loadings for the mothers' and fathers' Coping with Child (COPECHLD) scales are shown in Table 7.1. For mothers, the rotated four-factor matrix accounted for 53% of the total variance in the data for COPECHLD, 54% for COPESPOU, and 59% for SPOUCOPE. For fathers, the amount of explained variance was 54% for COPECHLD, 59% COPESPOU, and 58% SPOUCOPE. Items "busy self" and "yell/slam doors" displayed the weakest distinctions between factors.

The criterion for minimally acceptable factor loadings was a cutoff point of .30 (Nunnally & Bernstein, 1994). Based on factor loadings and content, each of the 13 items was assigned to one category. In this initial factoring procedure, no items were discarded. If an item loaded on only one factor, it was designated as belonging to the category represented by that factor. If an item loaded on more than one factor, irrespective of the relative loadings, the classification was determined by the nature of the items in the other category.

Scores for each factor subscale were obtained by summing the ratings for all items within the scale. Coefficient alphas for each subscale (and for the total scale) were obtained. The alpha coefficients ranged from .36 to .71; all but one was over .50. Because the number of items in each

TABLE 7.1 Four-Factor Solution of the CICI:PQ COPECHILD Scale for Mothers and Fathers

Coping strategy	Mothers[a]				Fathers[a]			
	1	2	3	4	1	2	3	4
Hide feelings	.75				.61			
Ignore/forget	.74				.70			
Busy self	.52		.42		.45		.51	
Get away	.51			.35	.60			
Take alcohol		.66						.68
Smoke		.62		−.41	.59			
Yell/slam doors		.61			.41	.33		
Take medicine		.54						.81
Cry			.74				.72	
Pray			.60				.72	
Exercise	.32			.69		.75	.30	
Ask for help			.38	.66			.72	
Talk with someone			.52	.55		.55	.40	
Eigenvalue	2.8	1.7	1.2	1.1	2.9	1.6	1.4	1.1
% Variance	21.7	13.4	9.4	8.6	22.6	12.1	10.7	8.3
Cumulative %	21.7	35.1	44.5	53.0	22.6	34.7	45.5	53.8
Alpha	.62	.50	.36	.57				

[a]Factor loadings above .30.

factor was small and many of the coefficients were low, further analyses to compare data based on the subscales were not conducted.

Criterion-Related Validity

As part of a study of parents of children with cystic fibrosis (Hymovich & Baker, 1985), data were collected from professional health care staff about how well the parents were coping. Data were available for 43 mothers These scores were correlated with the parent scores on the SElFCOPE (COPECHLD and COPESPOU) and SPOUCOPE scales to look at criterion-related validity. There was a significant correlation ($r = .28$, $p = .04$) for both scales using the Pearson product-moment correlation coefficient.

Item Level Results

Although results indicate general support for the preliminary validity and reliability of the Coping scale of the CICI:PQ, the coping items do not reflect the multidimensionality of the coping concept. Some of the items were skewed, and variability on some of the items was limited. For example, smoking, medicine, and alcohol were used by only about 25% of the parents. Although these items have limited variability, they were retained because of their clinical significance in helping parents cope with their child's illness. Also, deleting them from the scale reduced its reliability. In addition, highly skewed items and reduced variability can artificially deflate the alpha coefficient (Waltz, Strickland, & Lenz, 1991). Before these items are deleted, they should be tested in a wide range of situations so that frequency of item response can be compared. Modifications can then be made in a manner that will minimize the danger of deleting items that appear to have no value in a particular population or context but are, in fact, valuable in another.

The Coping scale of the CICI:PQ (COPECHLD, COPESPOU, SPOU-COPE) consists primarily of emotion-focused items. Only 2 of the 13 items are problem-focused. Emotion-focused coping has been found to be associated with studies of adults coping with physical illness and disabilities (Cohen & Lazarus, 1979; Lipowski, 1970; Moos, 1976). These studies show that much of the coping is directed toward managing feelings of anxiety, fear, and dread and toward restoring self-esteem and interpersonal relationships. It is possible that emotion-focused coping is more prevalent in parents of chronically ill children and that the parents and nurses reviewing the content validity of the CICI:PQ coping items responded to this prevalence. The instrument needs to be reviewed by experts in the area of coping rather than experts in the care of the chronically ill.

It was found that the format for the Coping scale was difficult for parents to complete because they must first identify whether or not the strategy is used, then how they changed its use. It is questionable how parents actually responded to these items.

Further refinement of the coping portion of the CICI:PQ was needed and was undertaken. A new instrument, the Parent Perception Inventory: Coping (PPICOPE), was developed based on this refinement process and is now ready for testing.

Description of the Parent Perception Inventory: Coping (PPICOPE)

The process used for developing the PPICOPE was that suggested by Waltz and colleagues (1991). Because coping is a multidimensional concept, the PPICOPE was developed to incorporate as many dimensions as appropriate. Additional coping strategies for the PPICOPE came from a secondary review of the parent interviews, from the coping literature, and from suggestions made by those who reviewed and used the instrument as it was being developed.

The coping items of the CICI:PQ were retained and incorporated into the PPICOPE. The PPICOPE is a norm-referenced measurement tool to differentiate between the number, types, and effectiveness of coping strategies reported by parents of chronically ill children. It is a self-report instrument, based on the assumption that perceptions of coping are a subjective phenomenon and can be measured only by self-report. Only one situation, coping with child-related problems, was retained for the revised scale. This was done to make the instrument more parsimonious. The child situation was selected for this instrument because there is evidence that the presence of a chronically ill child affects the parenting role to a greater extent than the marital role (Kazak & Marvin, 1984). Responses to the scale were changed to provide two interval-level scales rather than one ordinal-level scale. Instead of asking whether the item was used more than, less than, or the same as before, the frequency of use is assessed.

The number of items was increased from 13 to 29 to increase the scale reliability from .68 to .85. The PPICOPE has two separate scales: one to measure the degree to which each coping strategy is used (not at all, rarely, sometimes, often) and one to measure the degree of helpfulness of the strategies ("never helps" to "always helps") (see sample items in Hymovich's PPICOPE, Appendix 2). For each item, the respondent is asked to indicate whether the coping strategy has been used within the past 3 months. The 3-month time referent provides a sufficient length of time for a problem to be present and yet is short enough that the respondent is likely to recall the event. Completion of the PPICOPE usually requires about 10 to 15 minutes. The scales are scored by summing the values of each response, which result in two scores: a coping strategy score and an effectiveness score.

According to Lazarus (1975, 1977), the way a person appraises a situation has a strong effect on the coping strategies used. Therefore, an item is included to state the extent to which parents believe they have some control over the situation (problems related to child care). Other items have been included to obtain parent perceptions of their overall beliefs about how well they are coping (see Appendix 2).

CONCLUSIONS AND RECOMMENDATIONS

This study has described the psychometric properties of the Coping scale of the CICI:PQ. Four psychometric properties of the Coping scale were studied: (1) internal consistency reliability of the scale, (2) content validity, (3) construct validity using factor analysis, and (4) criterion validity. The reliability of the CICI:PQ was shown to be adequate but needs to be increased. There is also evidence for the content and construct validity of the instrument. Because a number of weaknesses were noted, a new instrument, the Parent Perception Inventory: Coping (PPICOPE), was constructed, using items from the CICI:PQ. This instrument is relevant to nursing practice.

In conclusion, a review of the psychometric properties of the CICI:PQ Coping scale indicated the need for a number of revisions. These revisions resulted in a new instrument, the PPICOPE. It is anticipated that this new instrument, which contains both problem- and emotion-focused items, will be useful to nurses who are trying to help parents adapt to their child's chronic illness.

ACKNOWLEDGEMENT

The author wishes to thank Dr. Carolyn Waltz, consultant on this project, as well as Dr. Ruth McCorkle and Dr. Barbara Munroe for their assistance in conducting the psychometric analysis. This study was partially supported by NIH grant T32 NR07036.

REFERENCES

Aldwin, C., Folkman, S., Schaefer, C., Coyne, J., & Lazarus, E. (1980, September). *Ways of coping checklist: A process measure.* Paper presented at the annual meeting of the American Psychological Association, Montreal.

Averill, J. R., & Opton, E. M., Jr. (1968). Psychophysiological assessment: Rationale and problems. In P. McReynolds (Ed.), *Advances in psychosocial assessment* (Vol. 1, pp. 265–268). Palo Alto, CA: Science and Behavior.

Burish, T. G., & Bradley, L. A. (1983). Coping with chronic disease: Definitions and issues. In T. G. Burish & L. A. Bradley (Eds.), *Coping with chronic disease* (pp. 3–12). New York: Academic Press.

Cohen, R., & Lazarus, R. S. (1979). Coping with the stresses of illness. In G. C. Stone, F. Cohen, & N. E. Adler (Eds.), *Health psychology: A handbook* (pp. 217–254). San Francisco: Josey-Bass.

Folkman, S., & Lazarus, R. S. (1980). An analysis of coping in a middle-aged community sample. *Journal of Health and Social Behavior, 21,* 219–239.

Folkman, S., Schaefer, C., & Lazarus, R. S. (1979). Cognitive processes as mediators of stress and coping. In V. Hamilton & D. M. Warburton (Eds.), *Human stress and cognition: An information processing approach* (pp. 265–298). London: Wiley.

Hymovich, D. P. (1981). Assessing the impact of chronic childhood illness on the family and parent coping. *Image, 13,* 71–74.

Hymovich, D. P. (1983). The chronicity impact and coping instrument: Parent questionnaire. *Nursing Research, 32,* 275–281.

Hymovich, D. P. (1984). Development of the chronicity impact and coping instrument: Parent questionnaire (CICI:PQ). *Nursing Research, 33,* 218–222.

Hymovich, D. P. (1987). Assessing families of children with cystic fibrosis. In L. M. Wright & M. Leahey (Eds.), *Families and chronic illness* (pp. 133–146). Springhouse, PA: Springhouse.

Hymovich, D. P. (1990). Measuring parental coping when a child is chronically ill. In O. L. Strickland & C. F. Waltz, (Eds.), *Measurement of nursing outcomes: Measuring client self-care and coping skills* (Vol. 4, pp. 96–117). New York: Springer Publishing Co.

Hymovich, D. P., & Baker, C. D. (1985). The needs, concerns and coping of parents of children with cystic fibrosis. *Family Relations, 34,* 91–97.

Kazak, A., & Marvin, R. (1984). Differences, difficulties, and adaptation: Stress and social networks in families with a handicapped child. *Family Relations, 33,* 66–67.

Lazarus, R. S. (1975). The self-regulation of emotion. In L. Levi (Ed.), *Emotions: Their parameters and measurement* (pp. 47–67). New York: Raven.

Lazarus, R. S. (1977). Cognitive and coping processes in emotion. In A. Monat & R. S. Lazarus (Eds.), *Stress and coping* (pp. 145–158). New York: Columbia University Press.

Lazarus, R. S., & Launier, R. (1978). Stress-related transactions between person and environment. In L. A. Pervin & M. Lewis (Eds.), *Perspectives in international psychology* (pp. 287–327). New York: Plenum.

Lipowski, Z. J. (1970). Physical illness, the individual and the coping process. *Psychiatry in Medicine, 1,* 91–102.

Moos, R. (1976). *Human adaptation: Coping with life crisis.* Washington, DC: Heath.

Nunnally, J. C., & Bernstein, I. H. (1994). *Psychometric theory* (3rd ed.). New York: McGraw-Hill.

Patterson, J. M., & McCubbin, H. I. (1983). Chronic illness: Family stress and coping. In C. R. Figley & H. I. McCubbin (Eds.), *Stress and the family: Coping with catastrophe* (Vol. 2, pp. 21–36). New York: Brunner/ Mazel.

Pearlin, L. I., & Schooler, C. (1978, March). The structure of coping. *Journal of Health and Social Behavior, 19,* 2–21.

Selye, H. L. (1976). *The stress of life* (rev. ed.). New York: McGraw-Hill.

Stewart, A. L. (1980, October). *Coping with serious illness: A conceptual overview.* Santa Monica, CA: Rand Corp.

Waltz, C. F., Strickland, O. L., & Lenz, E. R. (1991). *Measurement in nursing research* (2nd ed.). Philadelphia: F. A. Davis.

Weisman, A. D. (1984). *The coping capacity: On the nature of being moral.* New York: Human Sciences Press.

Weisman, A. D. & Worden, J. W. (1976–1977). The existential plight of cancer: Significance of the first 100 days. *International Journal of Psychiatry in Medicine, 7,* 1–15.

APPENDIX 1: COPING ITEMS FROM THE CICI:PQ

COPING*	Does not apply (1)	Do less (2)	Do about the same (3)	Do more (4)
Cry				
Busy self with other things				
Talk with someone				
Ignore/try to forget				
Hide feelings				
Get away				
Smoke				
Yell/scream/slam doors, etc.				
Exercise				
Ask for help				
Take alcohol				
Pray				
Take medicine				

*Additional stems for same coping items.

1. Parents handle their concerns in many different ways. There are times when you may have more problems or concerns because of your child's condition. In what ways do you do things differently when these problems come up? (Please put an "X" in the appropriate column. Do not mark on the lines.)
2. People do many different things when they become upset with their spouse. Please indicate the ways in which you do things differently when you are upset with your spouse than when you are not upset (Please put an X in the appropriate box. Do not mark on the lines.)
3. In what ways does your spouse do things differently when upset with you than when not upset? (Please put an X in the appropriate box. Do not mark on the lines.)

APPENDIX 2: HYMOVICH'S PPICOPE

Parents cope with their concerns in many different ways. There are times when you may have more problems or concerns because of your child's needs. The first column has a list of some ways people cope (manage their problems).

1. If you do not use a coping method in the list, circle the 0 in the first column.

2. The next three columns are choices about how often people do things to cope with (manage) problems related to their child's needs. Circle the number that shows how often you used the coping method in the past 3 months when you had a problem related to your child's needs.

3. The last four columns are choices about how helpful you find these ways of coping. Circle the number that reflects how helpful you find each of these ways of handling problems.

4. Leave the How Often and How Helpful sections blank if you do not use the coping method.

The format is as follows:

COPING	HOW OFTEN				HOW HELPFUL			
	(0) DO NOT DO THIS	(1) Very rarely	(2) Some- times	(3) Very often	(0) Never helps	(1) Some- times	(2) Almost always helps	(3) Always helps

Items added to the CICI:PQ

Look at options
Change my expectations
Ask questions
Use advice of others
Try to figure out what to do
Find help
Solve problem myself
Read about the problem
Wish problem would go away
Weigh choices
Get information
Try to change things

1. What have been your sources of information about your child's problems or needs? Check all that apply.
   ____ (1) clergy   ____ (9) social worker

____ (2) doctor	____ (10) nutritionist
____ (3) friend	____ (11) therapist
____ (4) nurse	____ (12) library
____ (5) teacher	____ (13) newspapers/magazines
____ (6) relatives or spouse	____ (14) support group
____ (7) pharmacist	____ (15) community agency
____ (8) other parents	____ (16) other _____

2. How often have you not known what to do when you needed information or help?

    ____ (1) never ____ (2) sometimes ____ (3) often ____ (4) always

3. In general, how well do you believe you are coping with problems related to your child's needs?

    ____ (0) not well ____ (1) fairly well ____ (2) very well

4. In general, how well do you believe you are coping with your feelings and concerns about your child?

    ____ (0) not well ____ (1) fairly well ____ (2) very well

5. Would you like us to help you with any problems you are having?

    ____ (1) no ____ (2) not sure ____ (3) yes

6. How satisfied are you with the way you are able to cope with the stresses you have?

    ____ (1) very dissatisfied   ____ (3) satisfied
    ____ (2) dissatisfied   ____ (4) very satisfied

Debra P. Hymovich © 1988

8

The Role Inventory

Marci Catanzaro

This chapter discusses the Role Inventory, an instrument that measures one's role identity associated with the social positions of parent, partner, and worker.

PURPOSE

The purpose of the Role Inventory is to measure role identity associated with the status positions of parent, worker, and partner. Role identity is the imaginative view that we devise for ourselves as occupants of particular social positions. The measurement of role identity involves the measurement of the meaning that an individual attaches to the role. The Role Inventory was originally designed for use with individuals with chronic illness (Catanzaro, 1982), but it can be used to assess role identity in general (see Role Inventory in Appendix).

Conceptual Basis of the Role Inventory

Role identity, a subunit of the global concept of self, is "the character and the role that an individual devises for [herself or] himself as an occupant of a particular social position" (McCall & Simmons, 1978, p. 65). Role identities are reciprocal relationships that are dependent on recurrent interactions between the person and others.

Mead (1934) suggested a relationship between self and role. The reality of self is phenomenological; to have a self is to view oneself from the standpoint of others with whom one interacts. Each of us has many selves, limited only by the number of others or categories of others who respond to us (James, 1910; Mead, 1934). In other words, self is the way in which we describe our relationships to others and is the result of our ability to evaluate our own behavior in terms of the response we believe the behavior would elicit in others (Stryker, 1964, 1980).

Identity is the subjective component of role. Identities are meanings we attribute to the self as an object in a social situation. These meanings of self become known and understood by us through interaction with others in situations in which others respond to us as performers in particular roles. The responses of others provide cues to appropriate role performance and, by implication, to a relevant identity for one who performs in suitable ways. The self is constituted from multiple and interrelated role identities.

PROCEDURES FOR DEVELOPMENT

Qualitative data obtained from 50 dyads, consisting of an individual living with progressive neurologic disease and his or her partner, were used to identify descriptors of role identity associated with the social positions of parent, partner, and worker. These descriptors served as the foundation for item construction of a norm-referenced semantic-differential instrument to index the connotative meaning of parent, partner, and worker. Adjectives used by the respondents were listed and duplicates eliminated.

The list of 140 adjectives was submitted to a panel of five parents, five workers, and five partners. Each was asked to judge (1) whether the adjectives could be used to describe their role in the three positions and (2) whether the content domain of the constructs had been adequately sampled. Two content experts in identity and identity measurement also evaluated the appropriateness of the adjectives. The 17 judges were asked to evaluate the adjectives and assign them a rating of "highly useful," "somewhat useful," or "not useful" to describe their roles. Judges also were asked to list other adjectives that would be useful in describing a parent, partner, or worker. No new adjectives were added.

DESCRIPTION

The 19 adjectives that were ranked "highly useful" by all 17 panel members formed the basis of a semantic-differential scale. The opposite adjectives that formed the bipolar pairs were selected for each word using the "Semantic Atlas for American English" (Snider & Osgood, 1969). The same list of bipolar adjectives was used to evaluate each of the three status positions. The directions at the top of each page were changed to reflect the concepts of parent, worker, or spouse/partner.

ADMINISTRATION AND SCORING

The scale is self-administered. Respondents are directed to place an *X* on the 5-point line between each pair of bipolar adjectives in the position that best describes themselves on each of three roles, that is, as parent, worker, and spouse/partner. Each concept is scored by converting the line between the bipolar adjectives to a numerical score, with the high values assigned to the positive adjective. Ratings are summed over all bipolar adjective pairs for each role concept. Scores for each bipolar adjective pair are calculated by assigning numbers ranging from 1 to 5, with 1 representing the negative adjective and 5 the positive adjective. Total role concept scores are obtained by summing the responses across all adjective pairs. Possible concept scores range from 19 to 95 for each concept, with high scores indicating a positive image of self in the role and low scores indicating a negative image of self. Scores for the concepts of worker, parent, and spouse/partner are calculated separately because each part of the Role Inventory is designed to be used independently of the others.

RELIABILITY AND VALIDITY EVIDENCE

Sample

The sample on which reliability and validity assessments were conducted included 232 (60.6%) women and 153 (39.4%) men. Among these were 77 single parents. The mean age of respondents was 42.5 years (SD = 7.5), with a range of 27 to 70 years. Ninety-seven percent (n = 370) of the respondents were Caucasian, with African Americans, Hispanics, Asian Americans, and Native Americans making up the remaining 3%. Nearly half (n = 173) had at least one college degree, including 4 with doctorates, 41 with master's degrees, 82 with bachelor's degrees, and 50 with associate degrees. Fourteen (3.7%) had not completed high school. Men and women with multiple sclerosis and their spouses completed the survey. The greatest percent of respondents were ill women and their husbands. Six single men and 71 single women also participated.

Reliability

Internal consistency was estimated with Cronbach's alpha, and with coefficient theta derived from the factor analysis.

Partner/Spouse Identity

The partner/spouse role identity concept questionnaire was completed by 307 individuals who were living with partners at the time of the study. The mean adjective scale score for spouse was 3.98 (SD = .33; median = 4; mode = 4). Total concept scores ranged from 40 to 95, with a scale mean of 70.99 (*SD* = 20.2). Internal consistency, estimated with Cronbach's alpha was .91. The theta coefficient was .87. Interitem correlations ranged from .06 to .67, with an average interitem correlation of 0.358. Item-to-scale correlations ranged from *r* = .37 to *r* = .69.

Worker Identity

The worker concept questionnaire was completed by 372 individuals. The Hollingshead (1965) Social Status Index was used to categorize occupations. Professional, manager, and sales personnel made up 38.5% of the sample, and the remainder consisted of clerical, craft, operative, service, laborers, and farm workers. Nine percent indicated no occupation. Full time employment was held by 176 (47.3%) respondents, and 43 (11.6%) were employed part time. The remaining 153 (41.1%) were retired or currently unemployed.

The mean adjective scale score for worker identity was 4.11 (*SD* = .39; median = 5; mode = 4). Cronbach's alpha was .90, and theta was .86. Total concept scores ranged from 46 to 95, with a scale mean of 74.62 (*SD* = 18.2). Interitem correlations ranged from .002 to .66, with an average interitem correlation of .34. Item-to-scale correlations ranged from *r* = .39 to *r* = .69.

Parent Identity

Parental status was claimed by 325 respondents. The mean number of children was 2.3, with a standard deviation of 1.02. The ages of children ranged from 1 to 46 years. The individual scale scores had a mean of 3.9 (*SD* = .42; median = 4; mode = 4). Total concept scores ranged from 42 to 95 (mean = 62.98; *SD* = 28.06). Cronbach's alpha internal consistency reliability was established for the concept of parent at .91. Coefficient theta was .85. Interitem correlations ranged from −.13 to .71, with an average interitem correlation of .31. Item-to-scale correlations ranged, from *r* = .25 to *r* = .64.

Validity

The manner in which the list of adjectives was derived provided a priori content validity of the role inventory. One hundred individuals were asked, during face-to-face interviews, to describe themselves as parents, as partners, and as workers. All 140 unique adjectives that were used in response to this open-ended question were listed and submitted to a panel of 17 judges. Only the 19 adjectives that were ranked by all 17 judges as "highly useful" to describe a parent, a partner, and a worker were retained.

Construct validity was assessed using exploratory factor analysis. Principal-components factor analysis with orthogonal varimax rotation was conducted. Only the responses of those participants were used who had responded to all 19 adjective pairs for the concept being analyzed. A three-factor solution was achieved for each of the concepts of partner, worker, and parent. This finding is consistent with the conceptual framework for the Role Inventory and with other authors' work with semantic differential measurement techniques (Osgood, 1962; Osgood, Suci, & Tannenbaum, 1957, Snider & Osgood, 1969). The evaluative factor was characterized by the items *good–bad, kind–cruel,* and *fair–unfair.* The potency factor was characterized by items like *strong–weak, brave–cowardly,* and *rugged–delicate.* The final factor, activity, which was independent of both evaluation and potency, was characterized by items like *calm–agitated, active–passive,* and *relaxed–tense.*

With the concept of partner/spouse, the *good–bad* item contributed 40.54% of the variance and had an eigenvalue of 7.70. This item also loaded on the evaluative and activity factors with a loading of .43 and .48, respectively. The two adjective pairs deep–shallow, and fresh–stale loaded above a level of .40 on the evaluative and potency factors. *Beautiful–ugly* loaded above .30 almost equally on all three factors. All other items had factor loadings between .51 and .77 on their respective factors.

The adjective pair *good–bad* explained 37.54% of the variance for the concept of worker and had an eigenvalue of 7.13. The adjectives *good–bad, beautiful–ugly,* and *deep–shallow,* loaded on both the evaluative and potency factors with factor loadings above .34. *Sacred–profane* loaded on both the evaluative and activity factors with loading of .43 and .41, respectively. Factor loadings for all other items for worker were between .54 and .83 on their respective factors.

The adjective pair *good–bad* had an eigenvalue of 6.68 with 35.16% of the variance for the concept of parent. The adjective pair *fresh–stale* loaded on the evaluative and potency factors with loadings of .47 and .46, respectively. The pairs *good–bad, beautiful–ugly,* and *valuable–worthless* loaded on all three factors with loadings between .24 and .47. All other factor loadings were between .51 and .84 on their respective factors. See Catanzaro (1990) for specific factors loadings for each item for each of the three role identities.

SUMMARY AND CONCLUSIONS

The variation in total scores on the Role Inventory among the concepts of worker, parent, and partner indicate that the respondents do not place the same connotative meaning on each of these status positions.

Alpha reliability coefficients were .90, .91, and .91 for worker, spouse/ partner, and parent, respectively. All of these reliability coefficients are above the criterion of .80, which is the minimum acceptable criterion specified by Nunnally and Berstein (1994). The alpha coefficient of worker could be raised slightly by deleting the adjective pair *rugged–delicate*, but deletion of this adjective pair has virtually no effect on the alpha coefficients for parent or partner. This word pair is one of four adjective pairs that loads consistently on the potency factor.

Factor analysis supported the theoretical constructs of evaluation, potency, and activity. However, the adjective pairs *good–bad* and *beautiful–ugly* loaded on at least two of the three factors. This finding varies from those of other investigators who have used semantic differential in which the word pair *good–bad* had high loadings on the evaluative factor (Osgood et al., 1957; Snider & Osgood, 1969).

Further testing of the Role Inventory needs to be done to assess whether the instrument can be used to assess change over time in role identity in the areas of working, living with a partner, and parenting that occur as a result of role transitions. The Role Inventory could be useful for assessing nursing intervention designed to prevent the development of a negative role identity following major role transitions in the lives of chronically ill and other middle-aged adults.

ACKNOWLEDGMENT

This project was supported in part by Grant No. BRSG S07 RR05758, awarded by the Biomedical Research Support Grant Program, Division of Research Resources, National Institutes of Health. The author acknowledges Dr. Clarann Weinert, Montana State University, for her support and material assistance in mailing the Role Inventory to participants in the Northwest Family Health Study.

REFERENCES

Catanzaro, M. (1982). *Shamefully different: A personal meaning of urinary bladder dysfunction. Dissertation Abstracts International, 42,* 4166A. (UMI No. DEO 82–04984).

Catanzaro, J. (1990). The Role Inventory: A tool to measure role identity. In O. L. Strickland & C. F. Waltz (Eds.), *Measurement of nursing outcomes: Measuring Client Self-Care and Coping Skills* (Vol. 4, pp. 147–158. New York: Springer Publishing Co.

Hollingshead, A. B. (1965). *Four factor index of social status.* Unpublished manuscript. Yale University, Department of Sociology, New Haven, CT.

James, W. (1910). *Psychology: The briefer course.* New York: Holt.

McCall, G. J., & Simmons, J. L. (1978). *Identities and interactions.* New York: Free Press.

Mead, G. H. (1934). *Mind, self, and society.* Chicago: University of Chicago.

Nunnally, J. C., & Bernstein, I. H. (1994). *Psychometric theory* (3rd ed.). New York: McGraw-Hill.

Osgood, C. E. (1962). Studies on the generality of affective meaning systems. *American Psychologist, 17,* 10–28

Osgood, C. E., Suci, G. J., & Tannenbaum, P. H. (1957). *The measurement of meaning.* Chicago: University of Illinois Press.

Snider, J. G., & Osgood, C. E. (1969). *Semantic differential technique: A sourcebook.* Chicago: Aldine.

Stryker, S. (1964). The interactional and situational approaches. In H. T. Christensen (Ed.), *Handbook of marriage and the family* (pp. 125–170). Chicago: Rand McNally.

Stryker, S. (1980). *Symbolic interactionism.* Menlow Park, CA: Benjamin/ Cummings.

APPENDIX: ROLE INVENTORY

In this section we would like you to describe yourself as a parent, worker, and partner. For each of these roles there is a list of 19 word pairs that are opposites. For each pair of words, please place an *X* on the line in the position that best describes you. For example, if you believe that you are an absolutely fair parent all of the time, you would mark the item:

FAIR: __X__: _____ : _____ : _____ : _____ :UNFAIR

On the other hand, if you are an unfair parent sometimes, you would mark the item:

FAIR: _____: _____ : _____ : __X__ : _____ :UNFAIR

Now use the list of words to describe yourself as a PARENT. If you have never been a parent, check here ____ and go to the next page.

PARENT

GOOD:	____:	____:	____:	____:	____ :BAD
BEAUTIFUL:	____:	____:	____:	____:	____ :UGLY
STRONG:	____:	____:	____:	____:	____ :WEAK
CLEAN:	____:	____:	____:	____:	____ :DIRTY
CALM:	____:	____:	____:	____:	____ :AGITATED
VALUABLE:	____:	____:	____:	____:	____ :WORTHLESS
KIND:	____:	____:	____:	____:	____ :CRUEL
DEEP:	____:	____:	____:	____:	____ :SHALLOW
PLEASANT:	____:	____:	____:	____:	____ :UNPLEASANT
HAPPY:	____:	____:	____:	____:	____ :SAD
SACRED:	____:	____:	____:	____:	____ :PROFANE
RELAXED:	____:	____:	____:	____:	____ :TENSE
BRAVE:	____:	____:	____:	____:	____ :COWARDLY
NICE:	____:	____:	____:	____:	____ :AWFUL
HONEST:	____:	____:	____:	____:	____ :DISHONEST
ACTIVE:	____:	____:	____:	____:	____ :PASSIVE
FRESH:	____:	____:	____:	____:	____ :STALE
FAST:	____:	____:	____:	____:	____ :SLOW
RUGGED:	____:	____:	____:	____:	____ :DELICATE

Note to Users of Instrument: The same list of bipolar adjectives is used to evaluate the status positions of partner and worker. Directions at the beginning of each list of adjectives should reflect the concept measured (i.e., parent, spouse/partner, or worker). The author holds the copyright on the Role Inventory. Permission for use may be obtained from Marci Catanzaro, Ph.D., University of Washington, Physiological Nursing SM-28, Seattle, WA 98195.

© Catanzaro, 1987.

9

The Women's Role Strain Inventory

Cecile A. Lengacher and Eric Sellers

This chapter discusses the Women's Role Strain Inventory, an instrument to measure role strain of women who are engaged in multiple roles.

PURPOSE

No role strain inventory has been developed that measures the characteristics of role strain of women with the multiple role obligations of being an employed worker, mother, spouse, and caregiver. The population for which the instrument was designed is for multiple-role women who are working. This chapter describes the theoretical basis, development, and psychometric evaluation of the Women's Role Strain Inventory (WRSI) and identifies the different populations assessed in research.

CONCEPTUAL FRAMEWORK

The theoretical framework for this inventory is based upon Goode's (1960) theory of role strain and Sieber's (1974) theory of role accumulation. Goode's theory originated from the work of Parsons and Shils (1962), Linton (1945), and Merton (1957). Goode presents the scarcity hypothesis in that the social structure creates overdemanding role obligations, resulting in role strain. This supports a major assumption that multiple role obligations can be a source of role strain. Goode believed that an individual faces many role demands and cannot meet all of them; therefore, role strain is a "normal" experience that everyone encounters. In general, Goode believes that an individual's whole role relationships are overdemanding.

In contrast to this "impairment orientation" is the role accumulation hypothesis, which proposes that multiple roles contribute to better health and focus on the rewards or privileges associated with multiple role involvement. Sieber's (1974) theory of role accumulation supports the assumptions that involvement in multiple roles allows for rewards and privileges, overall status security, resources for status enhancement and role performance, and enrichment of personality. Coser (1975), Marks (1977), Sieber (1974), and Thoits (1983) each emphasized how a multiple role lifestyle can lead to personal growth and development. These roles can provide a means to participate in society and provide monetary and nonmonetary rewards. Furthermore, resources can serve as buffer roles, providing positive rewards and satisfaction. Results of this involvement can be sources of stimulation, gratification, and social validation.

The literature supports positive and negative effects of role strain. Negative effects have been reported by Hall (1972) (home role as the major source of strain for college women); Hall and Gordon (1973), Coiner (1978), and Hall (1975) (pressures of working contribute to the stress of women), Gray (1983) (women experience strains between home and career); and Thoits (1983) (women with increased roles exhibit greater distress than men). Baruch and Barnett (1986) reported that the quality of the role was more important than the number of roles. W. A. Hall (1992), Simon (1992), and Meleis and Stevens (1992) examined the effects of marital and parental role strain on psychological distress. Waldron, Weiss, and Hughes (1998) found that employment had no beneficial effect for married women. O'Neil and Greenberger (1994), Haynes, Feinlieb, and Kannel (1980), Meleis and Stevens (1992), Veroff, Douvan, and Kulka (1981), and Noor (1996) examined the effects of responsibility and stress upon well-being or health. Healy (1997) and Lengacher, Sellers and Berarducci (2000) found that role strain had a negative relationship to engagement in health-promoting behaviors. It has been suggested that stress in multiple roles and inadequate support may contribute to immunosuppression and disease vulnerability (Thomas, 1997). Lengacher, Gonzalez, and Bennett (2000) found that relaxation/guided imagery decreased role strain for breast cancer patients.

Role strain related to faculty and students has been the focus of research in nursing education. Lengacher (1996) completed a theoretical and research analysis of 5 years of research in nursing education. Mobily (1991), Piscopo (1994), and Steele (1991) examined role strain of faculty. Hasselberg (2000), Home (1997), Lengacher (1993c), Lengacher (1993a), and Sherrod (1991) examined role strain of students. In contrast to negative effects, positive effects have been found related to multiple roles of women. Van Meter (1976) found that role conflict due to school could be compensated or overcome by the feeling of "adequacy" that accompanied being in school. Verbrugge (1983) and Sorenson and Verbrugge (1987) found that women with multiple roles tend to have better health. Social support from husbands, and children has been found to protect women engaged in multiple roles from stress (Belle, 1982; Berkove, 1979; Brown & Harris, 1978).

Supporting Goode's (1960) scarcity hypothesis and his theory on role strain, combined with Sieber's hypothesis of role accumulation, a definition of role strain emerged. Role strain in this inventory refers to a subjective experience that can be described as tension, a driving force, (which could be viewed as a positive or negative force), anxiety, or frustration that a woman may experience as a result of multiple demands placed on her or the demands by others. After factor analysis, three subscales were identified: (1) *role distress,* which refers to the adverse strain associated with multiple roles of working, family and significant others, and personal (supporting Goode's theory); (2) *role enhancement,* which refers to a positive response to multiple roles of working family and personal (supporting Sieber's theory of role accumulation); and (3) *role support,* which reflects the importance of support of family, friends, and children, and significant others. As the concept of role strain is systematically studied, the definition of role strain can be refined to include new knowledge of related factors, situations, and populations.

PROCEDURES FOR DEVELOPMENT AND DESCRIPTION

Instrument Design

Content Validity

A review of the literature revealed seven content areas related to role strain. Content validity was determined for the content areas and items. As summarized in Table 9.1, it was very high (.91).

Procedures Used to Delete Items

Coefficient alpha was used to determine the reliability of the piloted instrument. Five items that had low correlations (negative to .20) with the total test score were deleted, which increased the alpha reliability from .92 to .93. Overall, in the revised version, interitem correlations ranged from .24 to .69.

Using exploratory factor analysis with Varimax rotation, three factors emerged. After the first analysis was completed, one item from subscale 3 (Role Support) was deleted to increase the subscale alpha to .80. The overall mean for the scale was 116.73, and the standard deviation was 21.89. The resulting reliability evidence on the 44 items is summarized in Table 9.1. Table 9.1 lists eigenvalues, item loadings range for each item, and percent of variance accounted for by each factor.

TABLE 9.1 Citation, demographic, and reliability and validity information for use of the WRSI.

Study citation	Sample and characteristics	Reliability evidence	Validity evidence

Lengacher (1997)	*Sample size:* 445 women
	Sample characteristics:
	Mean age: 37.9, full-time workers: 82%
	The sample consisted of 14% minorities, RNs 98%, LPNs 2%
		Alpha:
		  Overall .93
		  Distress .89
		  Enhancement .86
		  Support .81
		Test-Retest:
		  Overall $r = .79$
		Interitem correlation:
		Overall
		  Mean = .22
		  Range = −.08–64
		Distress
		  Mean = .32
		  Range = .08–64
		Enhancement
		  Mean = .26
		  Range = −.01–59
		Support
		  Mean = .27
		  Range = .04–51
			Content validity:
			A priori:
			  Items were generated from the literature, 7 content areas were identified. Items were generated from the content areas.
			Posteriori:
			  Content areas had a CVI index of 1.0.
			  CVI for all 44 items
			  Mean = .91
			  Range = .33–1.0
			Factor Analysis:
			  Exploratory analysis identified the 3 factors used to form the subscales
			Eigen values:
			  Distress = 11.1
			  Enhancement = 3.25
			  Support = 2.35
			Loading range:
			  Distress .33–.73
			  Enhancement .30–.67
			  Support .32–.67

TABLE 9.1 (*continued*)

Study citation	Sample and characteristics	Reliability evidence	Validity evidence
Lengacher (1997) (*continued*)			*Percent of variance Accounted for:* Distress = 40 Enhancement = 10 Support = 7 Total = 57
Saengmook (1998)	*Sample size:* 144 women. *Sample characteristics:* First-time working women within 6 months postbirth after maternal leave. Mean age: 30.9 Mean hours employed per week: 42.2, 72.8% had a baccalaureate degree Infants age: in weeks mean: 18.4. Baby care hours per day mean: 10.4.	*Alpha:* Overall .86 Distress .74 Enhancement .80 Support .65 *Interitem correlation:* Overall Mean = .13 Range = -.27-.73 Distress Mean = .17 Range = -.16-.55 Enhancement Mean = .22 Range = -.12-.65 Support Mean = .14 Range = -.13-.72	*Content validity:* The content validity was confirmed by 7 Thai experts in the fields of women's health, psychology, and maternal and child health.

TABLE 9.1 (*continued*)

Study citation	Sample and characteristics	Reliability evidence	Validity evidence

Healy (1997)	*Sample size:* 71
	Sample characteristics: Women with Coronary artery disease, ages 28–83, mean 68.2. The mean score for awareness of coronary artery disease was 72 months. The majority were Caucasian (82%), with 4% Black, and 12% were Native American.
		Alpha:
		  Overall .95
		  Distress .91
		  Enhancement .89
		  Support .80
		Interitem correlation:
		Overall
		  Mean = .31
		  Range = −.64–1.00
		Distress
		  Mean = .40
		  Range = −.46–.91
		Enhancement
		  Mean = .36
		  Range = −.63–.90
		Support
		  Mean = .27
		  Range = −.48–1.00	

Light (1997)	*Sample size:* 87
	Sample characteristics: Women who were working and attending a university nursing program. Mean age: 41, with 67% em-
		Alpha:
		  Overall .92
		  Distress .83
		  Enhancement .81
		  Support .87	

TABLE 9.1 *(continued)*

Study citation	Sample and characteristics	Reliability evidence	Validity evidence

Light (1997) *(continued)*	ployed full time and 33% employed part-time.	*Interitem correlation:*
		Overall
		  Mean = .20
		  Range = −.24–.72
		Distress
		  Mean = .23
		  Range = −.14–.62
		Enhancement
		  Mean = .22
		  Range = −.15–.62
		Support
		  Mean = .36
		  Range = −.03–.65	

Lengacher, Gonzalez, & Bennett (2000)	*Sample size:* 19.
	Sample characteristics: Women diagnosed with breast cancer, mean age: 51.9, all were Caucasian.
		Alpha:
		  Overall .93
		  Distress .91
		  Enhancement .80
		  Support .79
		Test-retest:
		  Overall $r = .58$
		Interitem correlation:
		Overall
		  Mean = .22
		  Range = −.51–.89	

TABLE 9.1 (continued)

Study citation	Sample and characteristics	Reliability evidence	Validity evidence
		Distress	
		Mean = .40	
		Range = −.11–.87	
		Enhancement	
		Mean = .23	
		Range = −.43–.77	
		Support	
		Mean = .22	
		Range = −.35–.82	
Hasselberg (2000)	Sample size: 69	Alpha:	
	Sample characteristics:	Overall .92	
	Female associate degree nursing	Distress .87	
	students. Mean age: was 27.9	Enhancement .82	
	and 47% were Caucasian, 13%	Support .89	
	Black, 4.3% Asian, 1.4%	Interitem correlation:	
	American Indian, 5.8%	Overall	
	Hispanic.	Range = .13–.71	
		Distress	
		Range = .19–.74	
		Enhancement	
		Range = .21–.63	
		Support	
		Range = .21–.74	

TABLE 9.1 (continued)

Study citation	Sample and characteristics	Reliability evidence	Validity evidence
Beckie (2000)	*Sample size:* 93 *Sample characteristics:* Women recently having an acute cardiac event; mean age: 66.2, 91% were Caucasian, 4% African American, and 1% Asian.	*Alpha:* Overall .92 Distress .80 Enhancement .85 Support .87 *Interitem correlation:* Overall Mean = .23 Range = −.32–.80 Distress Mean = .22 Range = −.28–.80 Enhancement Mean = .28 Range = −.04–.75 Support Mean = .34 Range = .06–.72	
Berarducci (1999)	*Sample size:* 52 *Sample characteristics:* Female nursing students, mean age: 31.4, 79% Caucasian, 10% African	*Alpha:* Overall .90 Distress .80 Enhancement .79 Support .87	

TABLE 9.1 (*continued*)

Study citation	Sample and characteristics	Reliability evidence	Validity evidence
Berarducci (1999) (*continued*)	American, 4% Hispanic, 2% Asian, and 6% other.	*Interitem correlation:* Overall Mean = .18 Range = −.34–.81 Distress Mean = .20 Range = −.21–.60 Enhancement Mean = .21 Range = −.21–.68 Support Mean = .35 Range = .02–.81	
Birtel (2000)	*Sample size:* 33 *Sample characteristics:* Women who have a spouse and a child under 6 years of age in child care.	*Alpha:* Overall .92 Distress .86 Enhancement .88 Support .78 *Interitem correlation:* Overall Mean = .22 Range = −.48–.85 Distress Mean = .28 Range = −.25–.85	

TABLE 9.1 (*continued*)

Study citation	Sample and characteristics	Reliability evidence	Validity evidence

Birtel (2000) (*continued*)		Enhancement
		  Mean = .33
		  Range = −.43–.82
		Support
		  Mean = .21
		  Range = −.29–.83	

Lengacher & Martinez (2000)	*Sample size:* 52
	Sample characteristics:
	63% married, mean age: 36, 78% were employed full time, 50% preferred to speak Spanish.
		Alpha:
		  Overall .91
		Subscale mean scores:
		  Distress 5,
		  Enhancement 48
		  Support 30
		Interitem correlation:
		  Overall
		  Range = .05–.66.	

Berarducci (2000)	*Sample size:* 96
	Characteristics: Female working women, mean age: 45, ethnicity: 88% Caucasian, 5.2% African American, 5.2 Hispanic, 1% Native American, and 1% Asian.
		Alpha:
		  Overall .89
		  Distress .83
		  Enhancement .79
		  Support .74
		Interitem correlation:
		  Overall
		  Mean = .16
		  Range = −.30–.70	

TABLE 9.1 *(continued)*

Study citation	Sample and characteristics	Reliability evidence	Validity evidence

Berarducci (2000) *(continued)*		Distress
		  Mean = .27
		  Range = −.16–.70
		Enhancement
		  Mean = .21
		  Range = −.06–.64
		Support
		  Mean = .19
		  Range = .18–.50	

DESCRIPTION OF SUBSCALES

Sixteen items loaded on subscale 1 (Role Distress), indicating that there was adverse strain associated with multiple roles of working and family/significant others/personal. The item-to-scale correlations ranged from .08 to .64. The alpha was .89. Items in subscale one are 4, 12, 13, 15, 16, 24, 25, 27, 28, 29, 30, 33, 34, 35, 42, and 44.

Sixteen items loaded on subscale 2 (Role Enhancement), indicating a positive response to multiple roles of working, family, and personal. The item-to-scale correlations ranged from .01 to .59. The alpha was .86. Items in subscale two are 2, 3, 5, 8, 9, 10, 17, 19, 20, 26, 31, 32, 36, 37, 40, and 41.

Twelve items loaded on subscale three (Role Support), indicating the importance of support from family/friend/children and significant others. Item-to-scale correlations ranged from .04 to .51. The alpha coefficient was .81. Twelve items in subscale 3 are 1, 6, 7, 11, 14, 18, 21, 22, 23, 38, 39, and 43.

ADMINISTRATION AND SCORING

Fifty items were written related to the content areas (25 were designed as positive items related to role strain, and 25 were designed as negative items). A 5-point Likert rating scale with responses of *strongly agree, frequently agree, agree, disagree* or *strongly disagree* was used (See Appendix). The items were coded so that the higher the response number, the higher the role strain experienced by the person. Items then were randomly distributed using a table of random numbers. On the revised 44-item inventory there is a possible range from 0 to 220 points, with 0 indicating absolutely no role strain and 220 indicating complete role strain. The following specific items are reverse-scored: 2, 3, 7, 8, 9, 10, 11, 17, 19, 20, 22, 23, 26, 31, 32, 35, 36, 37, 38, 39, 40, and 41.

RELIABILITY AND VALIDITY ASSESSMENT

Table 9.1 provides summary information from studies that have subsequently used the instrument. Reliability evidence is provided for each study, and validity evidence is provided where available. By comparing the reliability evidence from the original study with the subsequent studies, as identified in Table 9.1, it is evident that the instrument cross-validates across populations. The instrument has been translated into Thai and Spanish, and both reliability and validity evidence compare reasonably well with the original study.

CONCLUSIONS/RECOMMENDATIONS

In summary, the internal consistency of the WRSI is adequate, resulting in high reliability coefficients for the total scale and subscales. The subscale alphas are quite high, across different populations, supporting the construct validity for the instrument. Content validity resulted in a content validity index of .91. Evidence of reliability was demonstrated through the use of coefficient alpha and through test-retest reliability.

Strong evidence for construct validity was determined by exploratory factor analysis, resulting in three subscales: Role Distress, Role Enhancement, and Role Support. Negative aspects of role strain or role distress support the theoretical framework of Goode (1960) in which he identified that a set of role obligations may cause conflicting demands and role strain. Positive aspects of role strain or role enhancement support the theoretical framework of Sieber (1974) and his role accumulation theory, in which a multiple-role lifestyle can be rewarding. Role support indicates the importance of support of family, friends, children, and significant others while maintaining multiple roles, an important factor to be considered (Belle, 1982; Berkove, 1979; Campaniello, 1988; Hall, 1972; and Van Meter, 1976).

The major limitation of the instrument is the need to complete additional reliability and validity studies. Additional factor analysis and reduction of the length of the inventory needs to be a major consideration, along with the collection of additional data on special populations. Translation of the instrument into Spanish has been completed, and testing is in process. The instrument is currently being tested on other ethnically diverse populations to determine reliability. It is important to consider role strain in relationship to women's health and use this instrument to examine relationships between role strain and particular illnesses. The present version of the instrument is designed to measure role strain of working women. Because roles of women in society are changing and are constantly being challenged, an instrument to measure general role strain in all women is in progress.

REFERENCES

Baruch, G. K. (1985). Women's involvement in multiple roles, role strain and psychological distress. *Journal of Personality and Social Psychology, 49*, 135–145.

Baruch, G., & Barnett, R. (1986). Role quality, multiple role involvement, and psychological well being of mid life women. *Journal of Personality and Social Psychology, 51*, 528–585.

Beckie, T. (2000). *Evaluation of role strain, perception of health, quality of life, hope and optimism in women after an acute cardiac event.* Unpublished manuscript.

Belle, D. (1982). The stress of caring: Women as providers of social support. In L. Goldberger & S. Bresnitz (Eds.), *Handbook of stress: Theoretical and clinical aspects* (pp. 496–505). New York: Free Press.

Berarducci, A. (1999). *Increasing Osteoporosis knowledge in preventive behaviors: Evaluation of a theory based intervention.* Unpublished manuscript.

Berarducci, A. (2000a). *Increasing osteoporosis knowledge in preventive behaviors: Evaluation of a theory based intervention.* Unpublished manuscript.

Berarducci, A. (2000b). *Effects of an osteoporosis preventative cognitive-behavioral intervention on knowledge, self-efficacy, role strain and intention in midlife women.* Unpublished doctoral dissertation, University of South Florida.

Berkove, G. F. (1979). Perceptions of husband support by returning women students. *Family Coordinator 28,* 451–457.

Birtel, A. (2000). *The relationship between role strain and role satisfaction: Testing the moderating impact of coping, locus of control and role salience.* Unpublished master's thesis, Virginia Commonwealth University, Richmond.

Brown, G., & Harris, T. (1978). *Social origins of depression: A study of psychiatric disorder in women.* New York: Free Press.

Campanello, J. (1988). When a professional nurse returns to school: A study of role conflict and well being of multiple role women. *Journal of Professional Nursing, 4*(1), 136–140.

Coiner, M. R. (1978). Employment and mother's emotional states: a psychological study of women reentering the work force. (Doctoral dissertation, Yale University, 1978). *Dissertation Abstracts International,* (University Microfilms No. 7915806).

Coser, R. L. (1975). The complexity of roles as a seedbed of individual autonomy. In L. A. Coser (Ed.), *The idea of social structure: Papers in honor of Robert K. Merton* (pp. 237–263). New York: Harcourt Brace Jovanovich.

Goode, W. J. (1960). A theory of role strain. *American Sociological Review, 25,* 483–496.

Gray, J. (1983). The married professional woman: An examination of her role conflicts and coping strategies. *Psychology of Women Quarterly, 7,* 235–243.

Hall, D. T. (1972). A model for coping with role conflict: The role behavior of college educated women. *Administrative Science Quarterly, 17,* 471–489.

Hall, D. T. (1975). Pressures from work, self, and home in the life stages of married women. *Journal of Vocational Behavior, 6,* 121–132.

Hall, D. T., & Gordon, F. E. (1973). Career choices of married women: Effects on conflict, role behavior and satisfaction. *Journal of Applied Psychology, 58,* 42–48.

Hall, W. A. (1992). Comparison of the experience of women and men in dual-earner families following the birth of their first infant. *IMAGE: Journal of Nursing Scholarship, 24*(1), 33–38.

Hasselberg, B. (2000). *Perceived stress, role strain and role involvement, predictors of academic achievement in associate degree female nursing students.* Unpublished doctoral dissertation, University of South Florida, Tampa.

Haynes, S. G., Feinleib, M., & Kannel, W. (1980). The relationship of psychosocial factors to coronary heart disease in the Framingham Study. *American Journal of Epidemiology, 3,* 37–58.

Healy, M. (1997). *The relationship between perceived stress and role strain to participation in health promoting behaviors in women with coronary artery disease.* Unpublished master's thesis, University of South Florida, Tampa.

Home, A. (1997). Learning the hard way: Role strain, stress, role demands, and support in multiple-role women students. *Journal of Social Work Education, 33,* 335–346.

Lengacher C. A. (1993a). The development of a predictive model for role strain. *Journal of Nursing Education, 32,* 301–306.

Lengacher, C. A. (1993b). Development and study of an instrument to measure role strain. *Journal of Nursing Education, 32,* 71–77.

Lengacher, C. A. (1993c). The development and study of a role strain inventory. *Journal of Nursing Education, 32,* 71–77.

Lengacher, C. A. (1996). Role strain, role stress, and anxiety in nursing education: Theoretical and research analysis from 1988–1995. In K. Stevens (Ed.), *Review of research in nursing education* (Vol. 6, pp.40–66). New York: National League for Nursing Press.

Lengacher, C. A. (1997). A reliability and validity study of the women's role strain inventory. *Journal of Nursing Measurement, 5,* 139–150.

Lengacher, C., Gonzalez, L., & Bennett, M. (2000). *The effects of relaxation/ guided imagery on role strain, depression, health promotion, locus of control, self-efficacy and stress, and immune function in breast cancer patients.* Unpublished manuscript.

Lengacher C. A., & Martinez, S. (2000). *Spanish translation of the women's role strain inventory.* Unpublished manuscript.

Lengacher, C. A., Sellers, E., & Berarducci, A. (2000). *Role Strain, depression and chronic health problems, predictors of health promoting behaviors.* Unpublished manuscript.

Light, K. (1977). *Humor as a coping strategy: Its relationship to role strain in women.* Unpublished master's thesis, University of South Florida, Tampa.

Linton, R. (1945). *The cultural background of personality.* New York: Appleton-Century-Crofts.

Marks, S. (1977). Multiple roles and role strain: Some notes on human energy, time and commitment. *American Psychological Review, 42,* 921–936.

Meleis, A., Norbeck, J., & Laffrey, S. (1989). Role integration and health among female clerical workers. *Research in Nursing and Health, 12, 355–364.*

Meleis, A., & Stevens, P. (1992). Women in clerical jobs: Spousal role satisfaction, stress and coping. *Women and Health, 18*(1), 23–40.

Merton, R. K. (1957). The roleset: Problems in sociological theory. *British Journal of Sociology, 8,* 106–120.

Mobily, P. R. (1991). An examination of role strain for university nurse faculty and its relation to socialization experiences and personal characteristics. *Journal of Nursing Education, 30,* 73–80.

Noor, N. M. (1996). Some demographic, personality, and role variables as correlates of women's well being. *Sex Roles, 34,* 603–620.

O'Neil, R., & Greenberger, E. (1994). Patterns of commitment to work and parenting: Implications for role strain. *Journal of Marriage and the Family, 56,* 101–118.

Parsons, T., & Shils, E. A. (Eds.). (1962). *Toward a general theory of action.* Cambridge, MA: Harvard University Press.

Piscopo, B. (1994). Organizational climate, communication, and role strain in clinical nursing faculty. *Journal of Professional Nursing, 10,* 113–119.

Saengmook, S. (1998). *Relationship among role strain, maternal role attainment, and selected demographic variables of working women who are first-time mothers in Thailand.* Unpublished doctoral dissertation, Catholic University of America, Washington, DC.

Sherrod, R. A. (1991). Obstetrical role strain for male nursing students. *Western Journal of Nursing Research, 13,* 492–502.

Sieber, S. (1974). Toward a theory of role accumulation. *American Psychological Review, 39,* 567–578.

Simon, R. W. (1992). Parental role strains, salience of parental identity and gender differences in psychological distress. *Journal of Health and Social Behavior, 33,* 25–35.

Sorenson, G., & Verbrugge, L. M. (1987). Women, work, and health. *Annual Review of Public Health, 8,* 235–251.

Steele, R. L. (1991). Attitudes about faculty practice, perceptions of role, and role strain. *Journal of Nursing Education, 30,* 15–22.

Thoits (1983, April). Multiple identities and psychological well being: A reformation and test of the social isolation hypotheses. *American, Sociological Research, 48,* 174–187.

Thomas, S. P. (1997). Distressing aspects of women's roles, vicarious stress, and health consequences. *Issues in Mental Health Nursing, 18,* 539–557.

Van meter, M. J. (1976). Role strain among married college women. *Dissertation Abstracts International, 37*(2), 1258. (UMI No. 7618683).

Verbrugge, L. (1983). Multiple roles and physical health of women and men. *Journal of Health and Social Behavior, 4*(3), 16–30.

Veroff, J., Douvan, E., & Kulka, R. (1981). *The inner American: A self-portrait from 1957–1976.* New York: Basic Books.

Waldron, I., Weiss, C. C., & Hughes, M. E. (1998). Interacting effects of multiple roles on women's health. *Journal of Health and Social Behavior, 39,* 216–236.

WORKING WOMEN'S ROLE STRAIN INVENTORY

Directions: The following are questions related to the role strain working women may experience. Role strain is the felt difficulty in meeting multiple role obligations.

Please indicate to what degree you agree or disagree with each of the statements below by **CIRCLING** the correct answer. **SA**—Strongly Agree / **FA**—Frequently Agree / **A**—Agree / **DA**—Disagree / **SD**—Strongly Disagree

		SA	FA	A	DA	SD
1	My family/significant others criticize me when I am unable to complete my household chores.	1	2	3	4	5
2	I am working to please myself.	1	2	3	4	5
3	I feel good about working, it makes me feel that I am improving myself.	1	2	3	4	5
4	I am often tired because of work and it is difficult to handle the strain.	1	2	3	4	5
5	I feel strain for not having time to do things with my family/significant others.	1	2	3	4	5
6	My husband/significant other is not emotionally supportive to my work.	1	2	3	4	5
7	My husband/significant other is emotionally supportive of my work.	1	2	3	4	5
8	I still participate in community activities that are important to me.	1	2	3	4	5
9	Having little personal time does not bother me.	1	2	3	4	5
10	I can manage my time for different roles: worker; personal; and family.	1	2	3	4	5
11	I have someone who shares the household tasks.	1	2	3	4	5
12	I have had more strains/difficult relationships with my family/children since I have been working.	1	2	3	4	5
13	I seem to be ill more often when I am working.	1	2	3	4	5
14	My family/friends do not give me emotional support.	1	2	3	4	5
15	I find myself unable to satisfactorily manage routine household tasks.	1	2	3	4	5
16	I have no special time for myself since I have worked.	1	2	3	4	5
17	My personal health is better when I am working.	1	2	3	4	5
18	I am working to please others.	1	2	3	4	5
19	I am able to manage adequate time for my family/significant others.	1	2	3	4	5

		SA	FA	A	DA	SD
20	I have adequate time to complete household tasks.	1	2	3	4	5
21	No one contributes to my household tasks which puts a burden on me.	1	2	3	4	5
22	My significant others decrease my role strain.	1	2	3	4	5
23	My family/friends are supportive of me when I am unable to complete my housework.	1	2	3	4	5
24	I do not seem to have time for all my roles: worker; personal; and family.	1	2	3	4	5
25	I find it exhausting to complete my household obligations in addition to working.	1	2	3	4	5
26	Completing my household and work obligations is not difficult.	1	2	3	4	5
27	I feel guilty about eliminating activities at church and in the community.	1	2	3	4	5
28	I do not have enough personal time.	1	2	3	4	5
29	I feel pressure from working, it does not make me feel I am improving myself.	1	2	3	4	5
30	I feel badly that I have eliminated community activities since I have so many obligations.	1	2	3	4	5
31	I have a satisfactory routine for completing household tasks.	1	2	3	4	5
32	My working role does not cause me strain.	1	2	3	4	5
33	My working role causes much strain for me.	1	2	3	4	5
34	My significant others increase my role strain.	1	2	3	4	5
35	My family/significant others do not make me feel guilty for having less time for them.	1	2	3	4	5
36	I am able to handle the additional strain of working.	1	2	3	4	5
37	I have maintained good relationships with my family/children since I have been working.	1	2	3	4	5
38	My family/friends give me much emotional support.	1	2	3	4	5
39	My family/children do not demand a lot of me when I have to bring work home from my job.	1	2	3	4	5
40	I make special time for myself since I have worked.	1	2	3	4	5
41	I have maintained my supports in church activities and in the community which helps my strain.	1	2	3	4	5
42	I do not have time to complete household tasks.	1	2	3	4	5
43	My family/children get much criticism because I am working.	1	2	3	4	5
44	My family/children do not decrease their demands on me when I have to bring work home from my job.	1	2	3	4	5

10

The Demands of Immigration Scale

Karen J. Aroian

This chapter presents the Demands of Immigration Scale, a measure of the personal demands associated with immigrating permanently to another country or locale.

PURPOSE

The Demands of Immigration (DI) scale measures demands associated with immigration, including loss, novelty, occupation, language, discrimination, and not feeling at home. The DI scale is appropriate for immigrants regardless of immigrant category (e.g., refugee, undocumented) as long as the intention is permanent residence in another locale. The resettlement location can be specified as any country or region. Although the DI scale has only been used with immigrants (i.e., people moving across international borders), the scale may be valid for measuring demands associated with internal migrations such as rural to urban or regional migrations.

CONCEPTUAL BASIS OF THE DEMANDS OF IMMIGRATION SCALE

The DI scale (see Appendix) is based on a transactive model of stress whereby subjective evaluations of undesirability define the presence of stress. There are six subscales, defined as follows: *Loss,* longing, unresolved attachment to, and preoccupation with people, places, and things in the homeland; (2) *Novelty,* newness, unfamiliarity or information deficits about simple or more complex tasks of living and norms of social interaction; (3) *Occupational adjustment,* or difficulty finding acceptable work, status demotion, and occupational handicaps; (4) *Language accommodation,* or the immigrant's subjective opinion of having a less than adequate command of English as it is spoken in the United States, including ability to be understood; (5) *Discrimination,* including active or subtle discrimination, such as the notion that immigrants do not belong in the

United States or deserve the same rights as the native born; and (6) *Not feeling at home,* or feeling like a stranger or a foreigner who is not part of the receiving country.

Based on the literature about immigrants' mental health and psychosocial adaptation, we had a number of theoretical expectations for the DI scale. DI scores will be (1) higher (an indication of greater demands) among older and more recent immigrants, (2) associated positively with depression and other negative affects, and (3) inversely related to coping resources such as resilience and mastery.

PROCEDURES FOR DEVELOPMENT

The content domain of the DI was identified by synthesizing findings from three iterative grounded theory studies with Polish, Irish, and former Soviet immigrants (Aroian, 1990, 1993, 1994). Although its initial use was with former Soviet immigrants, the intent was to develop a measure that would be relevant for more than one group. Interview data about immigrants' experiences were abstracted into concepts and categories reflecting aspects of immigration that were reported as having negative implications for emotional status. Case comparisons were made to examine variations in the demands experienced by each immigrant group. This process yielded the theoretical definitions described above for the six subscales.

A pool of potential DI items were written as indicators of loss, novelty, occupation, language, discrimination, and not feeling at home. The content relevance of the items was established using a team of four experts who were chosen according to their experience with Middle Eastern, Southeast Asian, Afghanistan, Polish, and Filipino immigrants. Only items that received a rating of 3 or above on a 4-point scale (ranging from *not relevant* (1) to *very relevant and succinct* (4)) by all four experts were retained. Sixty-seven items (11 to 12 items per hypothesized subscale) from an original pool of 89 items received ratings of 3 or above by all four experts. All six subscales received a rating of 4 and were retained as originally defined. Therefore, the content validity index (CVI) of the scale was 1.00.

Following content validation, a Russian-language version of the DI Scale was developed through translation and back-translation and field-tested with 19 former Soviet immigrants. Three ambiguously stated items were revised and a fourth misinterpreted item was dropped from the DI scale. The resulting DI scale contained 66 items.

A more parsimonious and psychometrically sound version of the DI scale was developed and validated in a sample of 1,647 former Soviet immigrants, who were randomly split into calibration and validation subsamples (n = 762 and 857, respectively). Thirty of the 66 items were eliminated after item analysis of data from the calibration subsample because the items did not meet the following psychometric criteria: high standard deviation (> 0.80), item-to-subscale and item-total correlations (>0.3), and item-item correlations (>.30 and <.70). After item analysis, confirmatory factor analysis (CFA) was used first to identify the best fitting factor model for the data from the calibration subsample, then to cross-validate the proposed factor model with data from the validation subsample. The best fit was obtained and cross-validated for a 23-item, 6-factor solution. Additional reliability and validity analyses with the calibration and validation subsamples included internal consistency reliability, test-retest reliability, and concurrent and discriminant validation. See Table 10.1 for the results of the psychometric evaluations. For greater description, see Aroian, Norris, Tran, and Schappler-Morris (1998).

DESCRIPTION

The DI scale contains 23 items. The Loss subscale is comprised of items 2, 10, 18, and 23. The Novelty subscale is comprised of items 4, 14, 16, and 22. The Occupation subscale is comprised of items 5, 6, 11, 19, and 21. The Language subscale is comprised of items 1, 8, and 12. The Discrimination subscale is comprised of items # 7, 9, 13, and 20. The Not at Home subscale is comprised of items 3, 15, and 17. All of the items are negatively worded and are preceded by a qualifying statement that specifies the United States as the resettlement location. However, the qualifying statement can be modified to include another location. Items are rated along a 6-point rating scale according to the amount of distress associated by each of the stated demands. The ratings range from *not at all* (1) to *very much* (6) distressed.

ADMINISTRATION AND SCORING

Written instructions ask respondents to rate the extent to which they have been distressed by each of the stated demands as it applies to their recent (within the last 3 months) personal experiences as immigrants. Subscale indices for each of the six DI dimensions can be calculated by summing item scores and dividing by the number of valid items for each subscale. To calculate a grand total score, the subscale scores are summed. High scores represent greater immigrant demands.

CONCLUSIONS AND RECOMMENDATIONS

Although more evaluation of the DI scale is needed, findings from the studies reported in Table 10.1 are promising. Nonetheless, additional

TABLE 10.1 Studies Supporting the Reliability and Validity of the Demands of Immigration Scale

Study citation	Sample and characteristics	Reliability evidence	Validity evidence
Aroian, Schappler-Morris, Neary, Spitzer, & Tran (1997)	*Sample size:* $N = 450$. *Characteristics:* Former Soviet immigrants to Israel. Mean age = 44.3 ($SD = 18.2$). Mean years in Israel = 3.72 ($SD = 1.21$). The majority were married (68%), Jewish (95.3%), female (52.9%), and had a minimum of a college degree (52.2%).		*Construct validity:* Demands of immigration will be inversely correlated with resilience as measured by the Resilience Scale (RS) (Wagnild & Young, 1993). *Findings:* Total and subscale scores on the RS correlated negatively with the DI ($r = -.23$ to $-.29$, $p \leq .001$).
Aroian, Norris, Patsdaughter, & Van Tran (1998)	*Sample size:* $N = 1647$. *Characteristics:* Former Soviet immigrants to the U.S. Mean age = 47.8 ($SD = 16.7$). Mean years in the U.S. = 3.80 ($SD = 4.44$). The majority were married (69.8%), Jewish (83.7%), female (57%), and had a minimum of a college degree (69.7%).		*Construct Validity:* Demands of immigration will be related to psychological distress and will provide more specific information than the mere passage of time in resettlement. *Findings:* Select DI subscales (Loss, Novelty, Language, Discrimination, and Not Feeling at Home) accounted for 15% of the variance in psychological distress (measured by

TABLE 10.1 (*continued*)

Study citation	Sample and characteristics	Reliability evidence	Validity evidence
Aroian, Norris, Patsdaughter, & Van Tran (1998) (*continued*)			Derogatis's (1992) Symptom Checklist-90-R) (SCL-90-R). DI scores were more strongly correlated with distress than were years in the U.S.
Aroian, Norris, Tran, & Schappler-Morris (1998)	*Sample size:* $N = 1647$, split into calibration and validation subsamples ($n = 792$ and $n = 857$, respectively).[a] *Characteristics:* Former Soviet immigrants to the U.S. Mean age = 47.7 ($SD = $ 16.4). Mean years in the U.S. = 3.6 ($SD = 4.3$). The majority were married (71.7%), Jewish (84.1%), female (56.7%), and had a minimum of a college degree (71.6%).	*Test-retest* (over a 3-week period): $r = $ .82–.87 for the six subscales and $r = $ .92 for the total scale. *Internal consistency:* alpha = .82–.88 for the six subscales and alpha = .94 for the total scale.	*A priori content validity:* Items were from qualitative studies with Polish, Irish, and former Soviet immigrants. *Posteriori content validity:* CVI = 1.00, ($p > $ .05). *Concurrent validity:* Demands of immigration will be correlated with depression and somatization as measured by the SCL-90-R (Derogatis, 1992). *Findings:* $r = $ .52 for depression and $r = $ .46 for somatization ($p < .0001$). *Discriminant validity:* Demands of immigration subscales scores will be higher among older immigrants and decrease for more long-standing immigrants.

TABLE 10.1 *(continued)*

Study citation	Sample and characteristics	Reliability evidence	Validity evidence
Aroian, Norris, Tran, & Schappler-Morris (1998) *(continued)*			*Findings:* DI subscale scores were significantly higher for older immigrants (multivariate F $(6,473) = 5.94, p \leq .0001$) and for more recent immigrants (multivariate F $(6,473) = 14.70, p \leq .0001$) with the exception that Occupation scores were not significantly different for young and older immigrants. *Confirmatory factor analysis:* Factor loadings ranged from .67–.88. Goodness of fit indices strongly supported the proposed 6-factor, 23-item factor model.
Aroian & Norris (2000c)	*Sample size:* $N = 450$. *Characteristics:* Former Soviet immigrants to Israel. Mean age $= 44.3$ ($SD = 18.2$). Mean years in Israel $= 3.72$ ($SD = 1.21$). The majority were married (68%), Jewish		*Construct validity:* Demands of immigration will increase the risk of depression as measured by the Symptom Checklist-90-R (SCL-90-R) (Derogatis, 1992).

TABLE 10.1 *(continued)*

Study citation	Sample and characteristics	Reliability evidence	Validity evidence
Aroian & Norris (2000c) *(continued)*	(95.3%), female (52.9%), and had a minimum of a college degree (52.2%).		*Findings:* An increase in demands of immigration increased the risk of being depressed by almost twofold (odds ratio = 1.83, $p < .0001$).
Aroian & Norris (2000a)	*Sample size:* $N = 468$. *Characteristics:* Former Soviet immigrants to the U.S. Mean age = 49.59 (SD = 16.45) Mean years in U.S. = 1.73 (SD = 1.26). The majority were married (72.4%), Jewish (80.5%), female (57.5%), and had a minimum of a college degree (69.9%).		*Construct validity:* Demands of immigration will predict depression (measured by the SCL-90-R; Derogatis, 1992) at 2-year follow-up. *Findings:* Novelty was the only immigration demand predictive of depression at 2-year follow-up (beta = .12, $p < .05$). Novelty explained an additional 2% of the variance in T2 depression.
Aroian & Norris (2000b)	*Sample size:* $N = 253$. *Characteristics:* Former Soviet immigrants to the U.S. Mean age at immigration = 49.76 (SD = 15.15). Mean		*Construct validity:* The pattern of change in DI scores will differ for 3 depression groups (depression lifted, remained

TABLE 10.1 (*continued*)

Study citation	Sample and characteristics	Reliability evidence	Validity evidence
Aroian & Norris (2000b) (*continued*)	years in U.S. 1.65 = (*SD* = 1.21). The majority were female (55.7%), Jewish (79.1%), married (70.8%), and had a minimum of a college degree (73.5%).		depressed, or became depressed). *Findings:* The group whose depression lifted (but not the groups who became or remained depressed) had a significant decrease in their DI scores (mean T1 DI score = 3.70 (*SD* = .87), mean T2 DI score = 2.67 (*SD* = 1.09), *p* < .001).
Van Tran (1997)[b]	*Sample size: N* = 349 *Characteristics:* Vietnamese immigrants to the U.S. Mean years in U.S. = 7 (*SD* = 5.22). Mean age = 38.76 (*SD* = 13.76). Mean years of education = 13.95 (*SD* = 6.17); 52.1% females.	*Internal Consistency:* Alpha = .91 for the total scale	*Construct validity:* DI scores will be positively associated with age and depression (as measured by the Center for Epidemiological Studies Depression (CES-D) Scale and inversely associated with years in the U.S. and mastery (measured by House's (1986) Mastery scale. *Findings:* DI scores were significantly correlated with age (*r* = .32, *p* < .0001), depression (*r* = .35, *p* < .0001), years in the

TABLE 10.1 (*continued*)

Study citation	Sample and characteristics	Reliability evidence	Validity evidence
Van Tran (1997) (*continued*)			U.S.($r = $ -.36, $p < .0001$), and mastery ($r = $ -.52, $p < .0001$).
Tsai (2000)[c]	*Sample size: N = 73.* *Sample characteristics:* Taiwanese-Chinese immigrants to the U.S. The majority were in the 41- to 50-year-old age category (38.4%), with 8.2% age 20 or younger and 2.7% age 71 or older, female (65.8%), sponsored by family (75.3%), and in the U.S. 9 years or less (39.7%).	*Test-retest* (over a 28-day range. Mean days = 15.76): $r = .71$ to .91 for the 6 subscales and $r = .89$ for the total scale. *Internal consistency:* alpha = .68–.90 for the 6 subscales and alpha = .92 for the total scale.	*Content validity:* Items not included in the original DI scale but reported as relevant included aspects of novelty related to the legal system and running a household. Another demand category was increased distance from the homeland. *Exploratory factor analysis:* The factor structure was similar to the original factor structure except that Novelty items and, to a lesser extent, loss items were dissipated across factors and Occupation and Language items loaded on one factor.

Note: Reliability and validity evidence is for the Russian-language version of the DI scale unless otherwise noted.
[a]Sample characteristics and reliability and validity evidence are similar for both subsamples but, because of space limitations, are reported here only for the validation sample.
[b]Vietnamese-language version of the DI scale.
[c]Chinese-language version of the DI scale.

studies are needed to clarify whether the content of the 23-item DI scale is comprehensive and performs similarly with other immigrant groups, including immigrants to countries other than the United States. The DI scale has been used mostly with Jewish immigrants from the former Soviet Union and immigrants to the United States. Jewish immigrants from the former Soviet Union are highly educated, primarily urban, and have resettled in ethnic enclaves. Demands of immigration may be different for immigrants with less education, immigrants of color, immigrants who are isolated from coethnics, and immigrants who have resettled in communities that are vastly different from their homeland (e.g., immigrants from rural areas or developing countries). On the other hand, experts with experience with diverse immigrant groups (e.g., experts on the Middle East and Southeast Asia) rated the content of the DI scale as highly relevant (Aroian, Norris, Tran, T. et al., 1998). The content of the DI scale was also fairly comprehensive when used with Chinese-Taiwanese immigrants (Tsai, 2000). Finally, good reliability and construct validity of the scale was supported with Chinese-Taiwanese and Vietnamese immigrants (Tsai, 2000; Tran, 1997).

Only one study investigated whether the initial factor structure established by Aroian, Norris, Patsdaughter, et al., (1998) with former Soviet immigrants was invariant for another immigrant group (Tsai, 2000). However, the sample for the replication study lacked sufficient statistical power for factor analysis ($N = 73$ for a 23-item scale). Thus, additional psychometric studies are needed to investigate invariance of the factor structure.

One existing problem with the DI scale is that the Occupation subscale typically has a moderate amount of systematic missing data. Although this subscale contains items that apply to employed as well as unemployed individuals, some unemployed immigrants (particularly those who were retired or not looking for work) did not complete all of the occupation items. In future research, it might be possible to address this problem by dropping the Occupation subscale from the analysis. In one study, scores from the Occupation and Novelty subscales were highly correlated, but Novelty was more predictive of psychological distress than was Occupation (Aroian et al., 1998).

REFERENCES

Aroian, K. J. (1990). A model of psychological adaptation to migration and resettlement. *Nursing Research, 39*(1), 5–10.

Aroian, K. J. (1993, June). *Extension and refinement of a model of psychological adaptation to migration and resettlement.* Paper presented at the Sigma Theta Tau International Research Congress, Madrid, Spain.

Aroian, K. J. (1994). [The experience of immigration among former Soviet immigrants]. Unpublished raw data.

Aroian, K. J., & Norris, A. E. (2000a). *Assessing risk for depression among immigrants at two-year follow-up.* Unpublished manuscript.

Aroian, K. J., & Norris, A. E. (2000b). *Depression trajectories among relatively recent immigrants.* Unpublished manuscript.

Aroian, K. J., & Norris, A. E. (2000c). Resilience, stress, and depression among Russian immigrants. *Western Journal of Nursing, 21*(1), 52–65.

Aroian, K. J., Norris, A., Patsdaughter, C. A., & Tran, T. V. (1998). Predicting psychological distress among former Soviet immigrants. *International Journal of Social Psychiatry, 44*(2), 284–294.

Aroian, K. J., Norris, A. E., Tran, T. V., & Schappler-Morris, N. (1998). Development and psychometric evaluation of the Demands of Immigration Scale. *Journal of Nursing Measurement, 6*(2), 175–194.

Aroian, K. J., Schappler-Morris, N., Neary, S., Spitzer, A., & Tran, T. V. (1997). Psychometric evaluation of a Russian language version of the Resilience Scale. *Journal of Nursing Measurement, 5*(2), 151–164.

Derogatis, L. R. (1992). SCL-90-R: Administration, scoring, and procedure manual II (2nd ed.). Towson, MD: Clinical Psychometrics Research.

Tran, T. V. (1997). *Measuring depression symptoms among Vietnamese-Americans* (Final Report to NIHM, R03 49462–01A4).

Tsai, J. (2000). *Cross-cultural use of the Demands of Immigration Scale with Taiwanese-Chinese immigrants.* Unpublished manuscript.

Wagnild, G. M., & Young, H. M. (1993). Development and psychometric evaluation of the Resilience Scale. *Journal of Nursing Measurement, 1*(2), 165–178.

APPENDIX: DEMANDS OF IMMIGRATION SCALE

Instructions:

Below are a series of statements expressing the difficulties confronted by immigrants. Evaluate each statement as it applies to your *recent (within the last 3 months)* personal experience as an immigrant, and circle the answer that best describes how upset or distressed you are about the experience described in the statement.

	Not at all				Very much	
In the U.S.:						
1. Americans have a hard time understanding my accent.	1	2	3	4	5	6
2. When I think of my past life, I feel emotional and sentimental.	1	2	3	4	5	6
3. Even though I live here, it does not feel like my country.	1	2	3	4	5	6
4. I need advice from people who are more experienced than me to know how to live here.	1	2	3	4	5	6
5. I am disadvantaged in getting a good job.	1	2	3	4	5	6
6. My work status is lower than it used to be.	1	2	3	4	5	6
7. As an immigrant, I am treated as a second class citizen.	1	2	3	4	5	6
8. I have difficulty doing ordinary things because of a language barrier.	1	2	3	4	5	6
9. Americans don't think I really belong in their country.	1	2	3	4	5	6
10. I miss the people I left behind in my original country.	1	2	3	4	5	6
11. I have fewer career opportunities than Americans.	1	2	3	4	5	6
12. Talking in English takes a lot of effort.	1	2	3	4	5	6
13. Americans treat me as an outsider.	1	2	3	4	5	6
14. I must learn how certain tasks are handled, such as renting an apartment.	1	2	3	4	5	6
15. I do not feel that this is my true home.	1	2	3	4	5	6

	Not at all					Very much
16. I have to depend on other people to show or teach me how things are done here.	1	2	3	4	5	6
17. I do not feel at home.	1	2	3	4	5	6
18. I feel sad when I think of special places back home.	1	2	3	4	5	6
19. I can not compete with Americans for work in my field.	1	2	3	4	5	6
20. People with foreign accents are treated with less respect.	1	2	3	4	5	6
21. The work credentials I had in my original country are not accepted.	1	2	3	4	5	6
22. I am always facing new situations and circumstances.	1	2	3	4	5	6
23. When I think of my original country, I get teary.	1	2	3	4	5	6

11

The Haber Level of Differentiation of Self Scale

Judith Haber

This chapter discusses the Haber Level of Differentiation of Self Scale, a measure of the degree to which a person maintains intellectual functioning as opposed to being controlled by emotional forces within relationship systems, particularly the family system.

PURPOSE

The purpose of the Haber Level of Differentiation of Self Scale (LDSS), is to measure specific aspects of the concept of differentiation of self, one of the eight concepts of the Bowen theory (Bowen, 1978). Differentiation of self, which can be viewed as an index of self-functioning, characterizes people according to the degree of differentiation or fusion between intellectual and emotional system functioning. The purpose of the LDSS is the assessment of intellectual and emotional system functioning of individuals within a family system.

CONCEPTUAL BASIS OF THE HABER LEVEL OF DIFFERENTIATION OF SELF SCALE

The LDSS is conceptually derived from Bowen's cornerstone concept, differentiation of self. Differentiation of self is the degree to which a person can maintain intellectual system functioning as opposed to being controlled by emotional forces within the relationship system. The well-differentiated person has a balance between intellectual and emotional system function and is characterized by emotional maturity. The most relevant patterns and characteristics of differentiation occur in contexts of family and other interpersonal relationships (Bowen, 1978).

A person's level of differentiation evolves out of the family relationship system, which creates an environment that either facilitates or inhibits movement in the direction of differentiation. A person's basic level of differentiation, which assumes a certain degree of undifferentiation in all people, is established by the time he or she leaves the family of origin. It exhibits itself most characteristically at times of anxiety and stress, especially chronic anxiety and negative stress, when emotional, social, or physical dysfunction is most apparent.

Bowen (1976a) proposes that although people at all levels of differentiation are vulnerable to anxiety and stress, those with higher levels of differentiation will have lower levels of dysfunction, especially during periods of chronic anxiety and stress that have a negative impact on the family system. This relates to Bowen's notion that people with higher levels of differentiation have fewer of life's problems; those that they do have tend to be less severe and are recovered from more quickly and completely.

As such, Bowen's (1976b, 1978) description of differentiation of self and its conceptual relationship to anxiety and stress bears a similarity to what has been described by stress theorists as protector-vulnerability factors or as moderator variables of stress (Johnson & Sarason, 1978, 1979; Lazarus, 1977; Sarason, Johnson, & Siegel, 1979). As stress and anxiety increase from low to high levels, an increase in the level of differentiation will tend to moderate the effects of stress.

PROCEDURES FOR DEVELOPMENT

The starting point for the development of the LDSS was the reanalysis of the 41-item Kear (1978) Differentiation of Self Scale (DOSS) that was further developed by Kim and Merrifield (1982). Their factor-analytic and reliability studies identified a 30-item instrument composed of five independent subscales, rather than the unidimensional scale that was proposed by Kear (1978). The Emotional Maturity (EM) and Emotional Dependency (ED) subscales of this instrument appeared to most accurately reflect Bowen's description of intellectual and emotional system functioning. However, these two subscales contained only six questions each and had psychometric problems. Therefore, a decision was made to use the 12 questions in the two subscales of Kear's tool as the basis for a larger item pool for the LDSS containing only two subscales, EM and ED. Additional items for each subscale were developed and organized based on characteristics of differentiation described by Bowen that related to intellectual and emotional system functioning. The categories for the EM subscale included values and beliefs, goals, cognitive versus emotional processes, I-positions, assessment of self, and expectations of others. The categories for the ED subscale included decision making, need for approval, need for security, response to group pressure, feelings about self, and problem-solving ability (Haber, 1984). The original item pool contained 100 items. The results of the pilot study of the 100-item tool yielded a 32-item LDSS with an EM subscale and an ED subscale. The data from subsequent construct validity studies indicated that the original subscale structure of the 32-item LDSS was not valid. Factor analysis demonstrated a factor-loading pattern consistent with a unidimensional structure. In two different factor analyses, 24 of the 32 LDSS items loaded on factor 1 (EM). As such, the LDSS has been revised as a 24-item, unidimensional scale. These findings will be discussed in detail in the "Reliability and Validity" section of this chapter.

DESCRIPTION

The LDSS is a 24-item scale with 4-point Likert-type items. It consists of declarative statements to which respondents indicate their agreement. Response categories range from 1 (*strongly disagree*) to 4 to (*strongly agree*).

ADMINISTRATION AND SCORING

The LDSS can be administered in either an individual or group setting. It takes approximately 15 to 20 minutes to complete. Subjects are instructed to answer each item according to how well it describes them. Response categories consist of numbers indicating *strongly disagree* (1), *disagree* (2), *agree* (3), and *strongly agree* (4). Responses indicating evidence of differentiation are scored in the above manner. The higher the total score, the higher the level of differentiation of self. Items 1–7, 9, 10, 12, 13–16, 18, 20, 21, 23, and 24 are direct-score questions. However, responses to items indicating lack of differentiation are reverse-scored. Items 8, 11, 17, 19, and 22 are reverse-scored. Scores for the LDSS can range from 24 to 96.

RELIABILITY AND VALIDITY EVIDENCE

The reliability and validity of the LDSS was assessed in three studies during the development of the LDSS (Haber, 1990).

Reliability

Study 1

The pilot study sample consisted of 257 volunteer subjects (151 female, 106 male) who were recruited from undergraduate and graduate classes

at urban and suburban universities and community colleges and through
personal contacts. Fifty-eight percent of the sample was female, 92% were
Caucasian, and 58% were married. The average age of females was 32.9
years; of males, 33.1 years. Several religious preferences were reported:
38.2% Catholic, 29.5% Jewish, 20.5% Protestant, and 11.4% representing
other religious preferences.

The 100 item scale was the focus of Study 1. Item-to-total correlations
were computed for the 50 items of each subscale (EM and ED). Items on
each subscale that correlated most highly (.30 or above) with the total
score were selected for consideration. The 19 questions that were selected for inclusion in the EM subscale yielded an alpha coefficient of .86.
The 13 questions selected for the ED subscale yielded an alpha coefficient of .83.

Study 2

The 32-item LDSS was administered to another volunteer sample of 168
married couples ($N = 336$) who completed the LDSS and two marital
assessment tools. The sample was similar to the pilot sample. All were
high school graduates, the majority having obtained some college education. Over 32% of the females and 45% of the males had attended graduate school, and 59% of females and 77% of males held professional
positions. Almost 99% of the sample were Caucasian. Average ages for
males and females were 34.6 years and 32.2 years, respectively. Coefficient
alpha was computed. The EM subscale yielded an alpha of .86; the ED
subscale, an alpha of .80.

Study 3

The 32-item LDSS, as well as the State-Trait Anxiety Inventory (Stai;
Spielberger, Gorsuch, & Lushene, 1970), the Life Experience Survey
(Sarason et al., 1979), and the Behavior Checklist (Gordon & Mooney,
1950), were administered to 372 volunteer subjects (240 female, 132
male). The racial composition of the sample included Caucasians
(83%), African Americans (10%), Hispanics (5.1%), and Asians (1.9%).
Educational levels were 14.1% high school graduates, 33% some college, 29% college graduates, and 23.9 % graduate study. The majority
had incomes below $40,000. Most were married (50.3%), with 35%
single, 6.6% separated or divorced, and 1.5% widowed. Subjects were
recruited from community groups, adult education classes, work settings, and community and four-year colleges to obtain a heterogeneous sample. The reliability of the LDSS was assessed using coefficient
alpha, which resulted in an alpha of .86 for the EM subscale and .83
for the ED subscale.

Validity

Study 1—Content Validity

During Study 1, the content validity of the pilot tool was assessed by a panel consisting of two family theoreticians and practitioners of family therapy and an expert in tool development. The judges determined that all of the items were representative of the content domain for differentiation.

Study 2—Construct Validity

A varimax rotated factor analysis was undertaken to evaluate the construct validity of the LDSS with the 336 respondents in Study 2. The findings indicated that 17 of 19 items from the EM subscale demonstrated a factor pattern loading of .40 or higher on factor 1. The two remaining EM items did not load significantly on either factor. Six of the 13 items from the ED subscale also loaded on factor 1. Five ED items loaded significantly on factor 2. Two items did not load significantly on either factor. The results suggest that factor 1 accounted for most of the common variance (80.4%). The factor-analytic data indicated that the LDSS may, in fact, represent a unidimensional construct. However, a decision regarding this issue was postponed until a third study, with a more heterogeneous sample, could be undertaken.

Study 3—Content Validity

Content validity of the LDSS was reassessed by using the content validity index (CVI). Two judges, both experts in the area of Bowen family theory and therapy, independently rated the relevance of each item to each subscale using a 4-point rating scale, ranging from *very relevant* to *not relevant*. The CVI for the EM subscale was 95; for the ED subscale, 92. This indicates a satisfactory level of content validity.

Study 3—Construct Validity

Construct validity was evaluated using hypothesis testing and factor analysis ($N = 372$). Three hypotheses were tested that reflected propositions related to the concept differentiation of self. Hypothesis 1 stated that there will be a negative relationship between differentiation of self and trait anxiety. Pearson correlation coefficients between the EM and ED subscales of the LDSS and the Trait Anxiety subscale of the STAI were both $r = -.52$, $p < .001$. Hypothesis 2 stated that there will be a negative relationship between differentiation of self and state anxiety. Pearson correlation coefficients between the EM and ED subscales of the LDSS and the State Anxiety subscale of the STAI were $r = -.43$ and $r = -.46$, $p < .001$, respectively. The results of tests for hypotheses 1 and 2 provide support for Bowen's proposition that the higher the level of differentiation of self, the lower the vulnerability to acute and chronic anxiety. Hypothesis 3 stated that there will be a negative relationship between differentiation of self and adult dysfunction. Pearson correlation coefficients between scores on the EM and ED subscales of the LDSS and the Behavior Checklist (BC) were $r = -.53$ and $r = -.42$, $p < .001$, respectively. These data provide support for the proposition that people with higher levels of differentiation are less vulnerable to psychological dysfunction.

A second varimax rotated factor analysis was undertaken. The findings indicated that 17 of 19 items from the EM subscale demonstrated a factor pattern loading of .40 or higher on factor 1. All 17 items were the same items that loaded on factor 1 in the previous factor analysis. The results suggest a marked stability in the factor structure of the LDSS. Again, factor 1 (EM) accounted for most of the common variance (82.1%). As a result of the consistent data pattern that emerged in the stage 2 and 3 factor analyses, a decision was made to revise the LDSS as a unidimensional, 24-item measurement tool. All items that loaded .40 or higher on factor 1 was retained for this tool. Item loadings on the new version of the LDSS ranged from .40 to .70. Additional data contributing to that decision was a high correlation, $r = .70$, $p < .001$, between the EM and ED subscales as well as a combined alpha coefficient of .91.

CONCLUSIONS AND RECOMMENDATIONS

The LDSS currently consists of a 24-item, unidimensional family assessment tool that accurately measures specific aspects of intellectual and emotional system functioning of the Bowen theory concept, differentiation of self. The LDSS has demonstrated evidence of internal consistency reliability, content validity, and construct validity.

A limitation of tool development has been the relatively homogeneous nature of the samples. As such, a recommendation for future tool development would include further testing of the LDSS using a probability sampling technique that includes a more diverse population. Another limitation of the studies to date is lack of a specific focus on dysfunctional families and families in crisis. Future studies could test the tool on clinical populations that include multiproblem families coping with chronic or catastrophic illness in a family member. Expansion of the data pool to include such populations would facilitate the conduct of variety of reliability and validity studies.

The LDSS is clinically relevant as an assessment tool for clinicians working with individuals and families. The LDSS provides an index of intellectual and emotional system functioning. Clients can complete the tool at the time of their initial visit, and the score can be used as baseline data for treatment planning and future evaluation.

REFERENCES

Bowen, M. (1976a). Family reaction to death. In P. Guerin (Ed.), *Family therapy: Theory and practice* (pp. 335–348). New York: Gardner Press.

Bowen, M. (1976b). Theory in the practice of psychotherapy. In P. Guerin (Ed.), *Family therapy: Theory and practice* (pp. 42–90). New York: Gardner Press.

Bowen, M. (1978). On the differentiation of self. In M. Bowen (Ed.), *Family therapy in clinical practice* (pp. 467–528). New York: Jason Aronson.

Gordon, L. V., & Mooney, R. L. (1950). *Mooney problem checklist, adult form.* New York: Psychological Corp.

Haber, J. (1984). The relationship between differentiation of self, complementary psychological need patterns, and marital conflict. *Dissertation Abstracts International, 45,* 2102-B. (UMI No. 800521–3042)

Haber, J. (1990). The Haber Level of Differentiation of Self Scale. In O. L. Strickland & C. F. Waltz (Eds.), *Measurement of nursing outcomes: Measuring client self-care and coping skills,* (Vol. 4, pp. 320–331). New York: Springer Publishing Co.

Johnson, J. H., & Sarason, 1. G. (1978). Life stress, depression and anxiety: Internal-external control as a moderator variable. *Journal of Psychosomatic Research, 22,* 205–208.

Johnson, J. H., & Sarason, I. G. (1979). Moderator variables in life stress research. In I. G. Sarason & C. D. Spielberger (Eds.), *Stress and anxiety* (Vol. 6, pp. 224–243). Washington, DC: Hemisphere.

Kear, J. (1978). Marital attraction and satisfaction as a function of differentiation of self. *Dissertation Abstracts International, 39,* 2505-B. (UMI No. 78–19, 970)

Kim, W. H., & Merrifield, P. (1982). *A differentiation of self scale.* Unpublished manuscript, New York University, New York.

Lazarus, R. S. (1977). Psychological stress and coping in adaptation and illness. In Z. J. Pipowski, D. R. Lipsitt, & P. C. Whybrow (Eds.), *Psychosomatic medicine* (pp. 383–401). New York: Oxford University Press.

Sarason, I. G., Johnson, J. H., & Siegel, J. M. (1979). Development of the Life Experiences Survey. In I. G. Sarason & C. D. Spielberger (Eds.), *Stress and anxiety* (Vol. 6, pp. 279–291). Washington, DC: Hemisphere.

Spielberger, C. D., Gorsuch, R. L., & Lushene, R. E. (1970). *Manual for the State Trait Anxiety Inventory.* Palo Alto, CA: Consulting Psychologists.

APPENDIX: THE HABER LDSS

Below you will find a set of statements followed by numbers from 1 to 4. Please read each statement carefully. After reading the statement, decide how well it describes you. If you strongly agree with a statement, circle 4. If, however, you strongly disagree with a statement, then circle 1. Use the other numbers next to the statements to indicate whether you agree (3) or disagree (2). There are no right or wrong answers. Answer as honestly as possible. Please read and *answer all items.*

	Strongly Disagree	Disagree	Agree	Strongly Agree
1. I will change my opinion more on the basis of new knowledge than on the basis of the opinions of others.	1	2	3	4
2. I am capable of helping myself when I am in a crisis.	1	2	3	4
3. When I have a problem that upsets me, I am still able to consider different options for solving the problem.	1	2	3	4
4. I do not find it difficult to disagree with the opinions of others.	1	2	3	4
5. My life is guided by a clear set of goals that I have established for myself.	1	2	3	4
6. I usually rely on myself for help when I have a problem, unless it is appropriate for me to seek the help of others.	1	2	3	4
7. I do not find group pressure hard to resist.	1	2	3	4
8. It is hard for me to set long-range goals for myself.	1	2	3	4
9. I can decide on my own whether or not I have done a good job.	1	2	3	4
10. I have a well-defined set of values and beliefs.	1	2	3	4
11. A lot of my energy goes into being what other people want me to be.	1	2	3	4
12. 1 prefer to maintain and defend my own position rather than conform to the majority.	1	2	3	4
13. I am emotionally mature.	1	2	3	4
14. My ability to make decisions is not greatly affected by the disapproval of others.	1	2	3	4

	Strongly Disagree	Disagree	Agree	Strongly Agree
15. My knowing that I have done a good job is more important than the praise of others.	1	2	3	4
16. I make decisions based on my own set of values and beliefs.	1	2	3	4
17. My decisions and actions are based on the approval I get from others.	1	2	3	4
18. My decisions are not easily influenced by group pressure.	1	2	3	4
19. I do not behave in a grown-up manner.	1	2	3	4
20. I am comfortable about my beliefs and values even when others challenge them.	1	2	3	4
21. What I expect of myself is more important than what other people expect of me.	1	2	3	4
22. I will change my opinions to avoid arguments with people.	1	2	3	4
23. When important decisions need to be made, I consider all possible options.	1	2	3	4
24. My own assessment of the job I have done is more important than the assessment of others.	1	2	3	4

12

Measuring Guarding as a Self-Care Management Process in Chronic Illness: The SCMP-G

Linda Corson Jones

This chapter discusses the SCMP—G, an instrument that measures guarding, a self-care management process that individuals use in managing illness self-care.

PURPOSE

The Self-Care Management Processes—Guarding (SCMP—G) has been developed after several years of work, beginning with the discovery of self-care management processes (SCMP) by Jones and Preuett (1986) and continuing with the validation of SCMP (Jones, Hill, Honer, & McDaniels, 1986) and delineation of characteristics of guarding (Huffman, 1987). Although further testing and development of the SCMP—G is needed, the inductive methodology—moving from the discovery of phenomena through qualitative research to further research validation of the phenomena and specification of empirical indicators to develop a measure—may be helpful to others investigating new phenomena of interest to nursing. The SCMP—G is designed to be useful in assessing guarding as an SCMP in chronic illness.

CONCEPTUAL BASIS

Self-care provides the broad conceptual framework for SCMP and development of an instrument to measure guarding. SCMP are adaptive behavioral, psychological, and cognitive mechanisms individuals use in performing a variety of illness self-care actions. Individuals have a repertoire of SCMP in coping with illness self-care, although they may use the processes to varying degrees. SCMP exist when individuals assume some responsibility for care of their illness and use mechanisms that make illness self-care more under-standable, acceptable, or integral to their life. SCMP is distinct from compliance with a professionally prescribed treatment regimen. Some individuals use SCMP to adhere to a prescribed regimen; others use SCMP in developing their own regimen or avoiding the prescribed regimen.

Guarding, one of the SCMP, refers to the process of maintaining vigilance over self, the illness, the treatment regimen, the delivery of care, and important relationships. Empirical indicators of guarding are being alert and watchful to control the illness or effects of the illness. Two types of guarding can be identified: self- and social guarding. Self-guarding refers to attempts to protect oneself, check on the progress of the illness, and exert control over the treatment regimen and delivery of care. Social guarding includes attempts by individuals to protect their social network members from the illness and the negative aspects of the illness.

Four critical elements of guarding have been identified: (1) perceived vulnerability, (2) perceived controllability, (3) self-absorption, and (4) a sense of obligation. A description of each critical element will be defined and illustrated with actual respondent quotations from the study by Jones and colleagues (1986).

Individuals who use guarding perceive that they or their social network are vulnerable to psychic, physical, and social threats. They also believe and act as though they have the power and the capability to prevent, curb, diminish, or stop illness-related threats.

Guarding is also a self-absorptive process. Individuals are acutely aware of and sensitive to both internal body and external cues. In addition, they carefully think about what they can or should do, whereas before their illness they conducted daily activities without much conscious decision making.

Individuals view guarding as essential to adjustment and sometimes survival. This sense of obligation is expressed with language indicating a sense of both "must" (requirement) and "now" (urgency).

The purpose of the SCMP-G is to determine the extent to which individuals use guarding in managing their chronic illness.

PROCEDURES FOR DEVELOPMENT

Although the process of guarding was confirmed and two types of guarding were identified during the validation study (Jones et al., 1986), the critical attributes of guarding had not been identified. Therefore, the first step in developing the tool consisted of delineating the characteristics of guarding. The data related to guarding from the study by Jones and colleagues (1986) were reexamined. From the literature on theory construction (Chenitz & Swanson, 1986; Glaser, 1978; Glaser & Strauss,

1967; Walker & Avant, 1983), the following questions were formulated and used to identify from the data the critical elements of guarding, as described above:

1. Under what conditions did individuals use guarding?
2. Under what conditions were individuals not able to use guarding?
3. In what context did guarding occur?
4. What were the consequences of using guarding?
5. What were the consequences of not using guarding?
6. What words or phrases referred to guarding?
7. What characteristics differentiated guarding from the other SCMP?

Development of an Item Pool

After the critical elements of guarding were identified, a blueprint was constructed to guide the development of items. The blueprint incorporated the characteristics of guarding and the two types of guarding. The number of items for the item pool was based on the need to write enough items for subscale scores of self- and social guarding (at least 10 items each) and possible item deletion in the stages of content validity testing and item analysis.

Data from the second SCMP study were used in developing items. Four guidelines were used in generating items. Items were generated that reflected each of the defining characteristics of guarding. In addition, only items applicable to a variety of chronic illnesses were included. Actual statements or phrases made by individuals in the study by Jones and colleagues (1986) were used as much as possible. Items were stated at a third-grade reading level, using brief, simple sentences or phrases of fewer than 15 words. A total of 65 items was initially written. Two subscales were developed, consisting of self-guarding and social guard-

TABLE 12.1 Blueprint for the SCMP-G

Critical Elements	Type	
	Self	Social
Vulnerability	3	4
Controllability	6	2
Self-absorption	5	5
Sense of obligation	6	4
Total items	20	15

TABLE 12.2 Means, Standard Deviations, and Alpha Coefficients of Modified SCMP-G and Subscales (*n* = 56)

Scale	Mean	SD	Alpha	No. of items
SCMP-G	120.41	10.40	.75	35
Self	74.39	7.36	.78	20
Social	46.02	7.59	.78	15

ing. Weak or questionable items were subsequently deleted from the item pool.

ADMINISTRATION AND SCORING

The SCMP-G (see Appendix) can be administered in either an individual or group setting, requiring about 15 to 20 minutes to complete. The SCMP-G has two subscales, consisting of self- (20 items) and social guarding (15 items). The Self-Guarding subscale includes items 2, 6, 8, 11, 15, 18, 19, 20, 22, 23, and 25–34. The Social Guarding subscale includes items 1, 3–5, 7, 9, 10, 12–14, 16, 17, 21, 24, and 35. The response format for both subscales consists of a 5-point Likert format ranging from 5 (*strongly agree*) to 1 (strongly disagree). Responses to items indicating lack of guarding are reverse-scored: items 3, 15, 19, and 28. The possible range of scores is 15 to 60 for the Social Guarding subscale and 20 to 80 for the Self-Guarding subscale. A high score indicates high use of guarding.

RELIABILITY AND VALIDITY

Content validity of the SCMP-G was determined through review by two panels of experts. First, eight experts who were clinical nurse-specialists or nurse-researchers in the area of chronic illness were provided with a packet of materials describing SCMP and the defining characteristics of guarding. They rated the SCMP-G on a 4-point relevance scale recommended by Lynn (1986). The SCMP-G was revised based on their ratings, comments, and recommendations. The panel of experts recommended deleting 6 items and changing the wording of 34 items. With the deletion of questionable items, the resulting content validity index was 1.00.

Next, a second panel of five experts assessed the revised 59-item SCMP-G for item-to-subscale congruence, using information describing the defining characteristics of guarding. The experts categorized the SCMP-G items according to whether items reflected self- or social guarding. This process reduced the SCMP-G from 59 items to 48 items. The item-to-subscale congruence index for the 48-item instrument was .92.

Testing of the SCMP-G occurred in two phases. During the first phase, the instrument was administered to seven adults with chronic illness to check readability of the instrument and clarity of the instructions, identifying items that were unclear or difficult to understand. The subjects found all items understandable. Minor changes were made in four items. During the second phase, the SCMP-G was tested for internal consistency. A total of 56 adults with chronic illnesses completed the SCMP-G and a set of demographic and illness background questions.

Individuals were recruited. from outpatient clinics and a diabetic education program in the Gulf Coast area of Mississippi and Louisiana. All subjects had been diagnosed with an illness of at least 6 months' duration that necessitated that they follow some type of treatment regimen. The sample consisted of 35 females and 21 males. The main ethnic identification was White; 51 were White and 5 Black. Subjects ranged in age from 26 to 84 years, with a mean of 58.5 years. Forty subjects were married, 10 were single, and 5 were widowed. A total of 44 had completed high school, and of these, 23 had completed at least 2 years of technical training or college. Subjects' family income ranged from less than $10,000 to $70,000 a year, with over 60% reporting incomes of less than $30,000. Although the majority of the subjects ($n = 30$) had diabetes, 17 subjects reported having diabetes and another major illness. Nine subjects reported having a chronic illness other than diabetes.

The time since diagnosis ranged from less than 1 year to 43 years. Only 5 subjects had had their illness for 1 year or less, and 38 individuals reported having had their illness for more than 6 years. Subjects rated the severity of their illnesses on a scale of 1 (*mild*) to 7 (*severely*), in comparison with other individuals with the same illness. Severity scores ranged from 1 to 7, with a mean of 4.09 and a standard deviation of 1.79.

The SCMP-G was refined through item analysis. During this step, items decreasing the reliability of the instrument through low correlations and items artificially inflating the internal consistency estimate because of item redundancy are identified (Hinshaw & Atwood, 1982; McIver & Carmines, 1981). Only items that demonstrated a large range of subject responses and had item-to-subscale and item-to-total correlations of .20 to .70 were retained. A total of 12 items were deleted (6 from each subscale) because item-to-subscale, item-to-total, and interitem correlations were below .20 (see Table 12.1).

The mean, standard deviation, alpha reliability coefficient, and number of items for the total SCMP-G and the Social Guarding and Self-Guarding subscales are reported in Table 12.2. Nunnally (1978) cited the reliability criterion level of .70 for new psychosocial instruments and .80

for mature scales. Both subscales exceeded the criterion level for new instruments.

The Self-Guarding and Social Guarding subscales were significantly positively related to the total SCMP-G scale. The two SCMP-G subscales, however, were slightly negatively correlated ($-.03$). This low correlation indicates that the two SCMP-G subscales are more or less statistically independent, sharing less than 10% of the common variance.

CONCLUSIONS AND RECOMMENDATIONS

Initial reliability testing provides beginning evidence of the psychometric properties of self- and social guarding. The internal consistency coefficients for self- and social guarding indicate an acceptable stability. The very low negative correlation between these two scales suggests that combining them is not fruitful and that the subscales should be used as separate measures of self- and social guarding.

A great deal of additional psychometric research is needed. Work is under way to establish the test-retest reliability and construct validity through factor analysis of the SCMP-G. Further testing of the SCMP-G is critical for future research of guarding.

Several areas of inquiry concerning guarding seem particularly promising. For example, further exploration of the antecedents and consequences of guarding is needed. The study by Jones and colleagues (1986) revealed that the vigilant monitoring and controlling nature of guarding requires a great deal of self-investment and mobilization of energy. Some individuals spoke of not being able to "police" their treatment or of "losing control" at times. These instances of "failed" guarding were most evident when individuals were very ill and lacked the energy to invest in guarding or when threats were perceived as too unpredictable or difficult to control. The number of instances of guarding was much higher for some individuals than for others with the same illness. Do individuals who exhibit high guarding overestimate potential harm from threats? Although some amount of guarding may help, the consequences of using too much guarding may exact a severe energy cost.

Self- and social guarding appear to serve different functions. Whereas some individuals in the study by Jones and colleagues (1986) used both types of guarding, others used little social guarding. Does low use of social guarding result in high stress within the social network, eventually leading to low levels of social support being offered to the chronically ill individual? Conversely, does the use of social guarding protect the network from stress, thereby helping the network maintain the ability to return social support over a long period of time to the individual with chronic illness? Serious programmatic research efforts, as described in this chapter, are needed to advance clinical nursing knowledge.

REFERENCES

Chenitz, W. C., & Swanson, J. M. (1986). *From practice to grounded theory: Qualitative research in nursing.* Menlo Park, CA: Addison-Wesley.

Glaser, B. (1978). *Theoretical sensitivity.* Mill Valley, CA: Sociology Press.

Glaser, B., & Strauss, A. (1967). *The discovery of grounded theory: Strategies for qualitative research.* Chicago: Aldine.

Hinshaw, A. S., & Atwood, J. R. (1982). A patient satisfaction instrument: Precision by replication. *Nursing Research, 31,* 170–175, 191.

Huffman, D. M. (1987). *Development of an instrument to measure use of self-care management processes-guarding (SCMP-G).* Unpublished master's thesis, Louisiana State University Medical Center, New Orleans.

Jones, L. C. (1988). Measuring guarding: A self care management process used by individuals with chronic illness. In C. F. Waltz & O. L. Strickland (Eds.), *Measurement of nursing outcomes* (pp. 58–75). New York: Springer Publishing Co.

Jones, L. C., Hill, K. Honer, K., & McDaniels, S. (1986). *Self-care management processes used by individuals with chronic illness.* Unpublished manuscript.

Jones, L. C., & Preuett, S. (1986). Self-care activities and processes used by hemodialysis patients. *American Nephrology Nurses Association Journal, 13,* 73–79.

Lynn, M. R. (1986). Determination and quantification of content validity. *Nursing Research, 35,* 382–385.

McIver, J. P., & Carmines, E. G. (1981). *Unidimensional scaling.* Beverly Hills, CA: Sage.

Nunnally J. C. (1978). *Psychometric theory.* New York: McGraw-Hill.

O'Brien, M. E. (1984). *The courage to survive: The life career of the chronic dialysis patient.* New York: Grune & Stratton.

Walker, L. O., & Avant, K. C. (1983). *Strategies for theory construction in nursing.* Norwalk, CT: Appleton-Century-Crofts.

APPENDIX: SCMP-G QUESTIONNAIRE

Directions:

An illness may require many changes in your life. The purpose of these questions is to find out how different people deal with their illness.

There are no right or wrong answers. For each statement, circle the answer that best describes your thoughts. Please answer all questions.

	Strongly disagree				Strongly agree
1. I worry about being a bother because of my illness.	1	2	3	4	5
2. I have made up my mind that I can control my illness.	1	2	3	4	5
3. My illness does not affect my family and friends.	1	2	3	4	5
4. Pleasing other people is more important than my health.	1	2	3	4	5
5. I worry that I am a bother to other people.	1	2	3	4	5
6. I must do all I can to control my illness.	1	2	3	4	5
7. I am responsible for making sure my illness does not worry other people	1	2	3	4	5
8. I have to be careful with the way I live my life.	1	2	3	4	5
9. My illness has affected my relationships with friends.	1	2	3	4	5
10. I don't do certain things, because then people would worry about my health.	1	2	3	4	5
11. I worry that if I don't follow my treatment plan, my illness will worsen.	1	2	3	4	5
12. I am troubled that people treat me differently because of my illness.	1	2	3	4	5
13. Even though I think a lot about my illness, I try not to talk about it.	1	2	3	4	5
14. I try to convince other people to change the way they live so they won't develop my health problems.	1	2	3	4	5
15. It is hard to plan activities, because I never know whether my illness will keep me from doing things.	1	2	3	4	5
16. I must have a positive attitude about my illness for the sake of others.	1	2	3	4	5
17. My illness makes other people uncomfortable.	1	2	3	4	5
18. I only think about my illness when it causes me problems.	1	2	3	4	5
19. I don't think about my illness as I do daily activities.	1	2	3	4	5
20. I have changes the way I live to improve my health.	1	2	3	4	5
21. I tell people about my illness so they will understand if I'm out of sorts and they won't take it personally.	1	2	3	4	5
22. I can control my illness if I follow my treatment plan.	1	2	3	4	5
23. If I take care of myself, I can prevent further problems with my illness.	1	2	3	4	5
24. I am careful about how much I tell other people about my illness, because I don't want to trouble them.	1	2	3	4	5

	Strongly disagree				Strongly agree
25. I check myself for signs that my illness is changing.	1	2	3	4	5
26. When I make daily plans, I think about my illness.	1	2	3	4	5
27. I watch for signs that my illness is getting worse.	1	2	3	4	5
28. There is little I can do to control my illness.	1	2	3	4	5
29. I think about my health a great deal.	1	2	3	4	5
30. It is important to follow a routine so I can lead a normal life.	1	2	3	4	5
31. I manage my illness by learning all I can about it.	1	2	3	4	5
32. I have changed the way I live so that I can control my illness.	1	2	3	4	5
33. My life resolves around my treatment plan.	1	2	3	4	5
34. I must watch my health or it will get worse.	1	2	3	4	5
35. I go out of my way to make people feel comfortable with my illness.	1	2	3	4	5

PART III
Social Support and Quality of Life

13

Measuring Social Support: PRQ2000

Clarann Weinert

This chapter discusses the Personal Resource Questionnaire, a measure of social support.

PURPOSE

Social support is an intuitive and ubiquitous concept. Exploration of social networks can be traced to foundational work by Cooley (1902), Mead (1934), Simmel (1908/1950), and Moreno (1934). The dramatic findings of Nuckholls, Cassell, and Kaplan (1972), regarding relationship of high stress/low psychosocial assets and negative pregnancy outcomes, sparked further interest in the health-related nature of social support. As the role of social support in health began to be recognized and examined, an emerging theme was that the "human climate" played a significant role in maintenance of health and response to stress. By the early 1980's, nurse-developed measures of social support reached the literature. The initial developmental efforts on the Personal Resource Questionnaire (Brandt & Weinert, 1981) and on the Norbeck Social Support Questionnaire (Norbeck, Lindsey, & Carrieri, 1981) were reported in *Nursing Research*.

In her comprehensive review of social support, Wortman (1984) noted that although the nature, meaning, and measurement of the concept are still debated, social support has been claimed to have positive effects on a wide scope of outcomes, including physical health, mental well-being, and social functioning. Today there are still debates on and multiple definitions of social support. Likewise, there are wide discrepancies in the approaches taken to measure social support. Yet there are common threads of agreement: that social support has a positive influence on the experience of dealing with illness (Stewart, 1993); that, over the course of a long-term illness, individuals express the need for and describe the importance of social support (Irvine, Brown, Crooks, Roberts, & Browne, 1991); that social support has a positive influence on illness management and that support from others who have experienced similar health problems is of particular benefit (Helgeson & Cohen, 1996; Stewart, 1993; Thorne, 1993; Weinert, 2000); and that inadequate social support is related to increased depression in people with chronic conditions (Connell, Wayne, Gallant, & Sharpe, 1994; Faucett, 1994).

The Personal Resource Questionnaire (PRQ), a first-generation nursing measure of social support, was developed in the late 1970s. After its initial use in dissertation research, minor revisions were made that produced the PRQ82. The Measurement of Clinical and Educational Nursing Outcomes Project allowed for systematic revisions resulting in another revision, the PRQ85 (Weinert, 1988). Clearly, social support remains a key variable in nursing research, but it was anticipated that, as newer measures were developed and tested, enthusiasm for the PRQ would wane. This expectation was unfounded because requests for its use continue to come from across the global nursing community. The sustained interest in the scale, questions posed by researchers using the tool, and further research by the tool's developers encouraged further psychometric testing. The purpose of this chapter is to report the recent psychometric evaluation and modifications of the instrument and to present the latest version, the PRQ2000. Despite the continuing definitional and measurement debates, social support remains a salient factor in nursing research and clinical practice.

CONCEPTUAL FRAMEWORK

The Personal Resource Questionnaire (PRQ) (Brandt & Weinert, 1981) was designed using a synthesis of ideas based primarily on the model by Weiss (1969, 1974) of relational functions. Social support was defined as a composite concept including (1) attachment/intimacy, (2) social integration, (3) nurturance, (4) reassurance of worth, and (5) availability of assistance. The PRQ is a two-part norm-referenced instrument. Part 1 was designed to gather descriptive information on the social network and consists of 10 life situations in which one could be expected to need assistance. Based on Weiss's dimensions, Part 2 is a 25-item, 7-point Likert scale designed to assess the perceived level of social support. Five items were written for each of the five underlying hypothetical Weiss dimensions. Scores on Part 2 range from 25 to 175, with higher scores indicating higher levels of social support. The instrument is self-administered and requires approximately 15 minutes to complete.

The instrument has systematically and consistently undergone psychometric evaluation over the past 20 years, resulting in the PRQ82, PRQ85, and now the PRQ2000. The developmental history and psychometric evaluation are chronicled in a series of publications (Brandt & Weinert, 1981; Tilden & Weinert, 1987; Weinert, 1984, 1987, 1988; Weinert & Brandt, 1987), and information is kept current at www.montana.edu/cweinert.

The PRQ has enjoyed a wide circulation with application in multiple types of research projects. To date, 1,375 requests to use the instrument have been received, coming from every state in the United States, 9 Canadian provinces, and 33 other countries. The number of requests ranged from 17 in 1983 to 149 in 1989, with 28 requests thus far in 2002. The measure has been translated into six languages: Japanese, Chinese, Dutch, Spanish, Korean, and Thai. Those requesting the PRQ were nursing students (baccalaureate: 6%; masters: 41%; doctoral: 17%), nursing faculty (19%), and nurses in practice/other disciplines (16%). A computer database on user requests is maintained, as well as a file of all data provided by researchers, articles in which the tool was cited, and copies of the translations.

PROCEDURE FOR DEVELOPMENT OF THE PRQ2000

Earlier psychometric evaluation of the Personal Resource Questionnaire gave evidence that the five hypothetical underlying dimensions did not reflect the true dimension of the scale (Weinert, 1987, 1988). Likewise, several weak items were identified that did not factor cleanly, were not highly correlated with the other items, or were not strongly correlated with the total. These initial impressions were presented by Weinert (1987, 1988) with caveats about the use of pooled data sets in order to build an adequate sample for psychometric evaluation of an instrument.

As an adequate sample became available, further examination of the psychometric properties was possible. The evaluation of the multidimensionality of Part 2 was conducted using the same techniques employed earlier and described in detail by Weinert (1987, 1988). A sample of 899 participants was used from the Family Health Study, a nation-wide study of families managing multiple sclerosis. Data had been collected from middlecent participants in 47 states using a mail questionnaire. Cronbach's alpha for the PRQ85 for the total sample was .92, which is consistent with alphas reported across multiple studies (Table 13.1). The Family Health Study data set was randomly divided into two: sub-sample 1 ($N = 449$) and sub-sample 2 ($N = 450$). The alpha for sub-sample 1 was .93 and the alpha for sub-sample 2 was .91.

Sub-sample 1 Analysis

In the earlier factor analysis (Weinert, 1987, 1988), Rao's factoring was selected, because it was designed to find a factor solution in which the correlation between the hypothesized factors and the set of data variables were maximized. Likewise, oblique rotation was used to allow the initial factor to rotate to best summarize any clustering of variables, and factors were allowed to correlate if such correlations existed in the data.

TABLE 13.1 Sample of Studies in Which the PRQ85 Was Used

Study	Sample	Alpha
Family Health Study—Time 1	National sample of couples (mean age: 45.5) living with multiple sclerosis ($N = 722$)	.91
Family Health Study—Time 2	National sample of couples (mean age: 44.5) living with multiple sclerosis ($N = 1,204$)	.92
Family Health Study—Time 3	National sample of couples (mean age: 46.5 living with multiple sclerosis ($N = 1,157$)	.92
Family Health Study—Time 4	National sample of couples (mean age: 47.3) living with multiple sclerosis ($N = 1,058$)	.91
Montana Family Cancer Project—T1	Montana and Northern Wyoming persons with cancer and their caregivers (mean age: 58.7) ($N = 840$)	.76
Montana Family Cancer Project—T2	Montana and Northern Wyoming persons with cancer and their caregivers (mean age: 59.2) ($N = 588$)	.80
Montana Family Survey	Rural Montana, Wyoming, Washington, North Dakota men and women (mean age: 46.8) ($N = 302$)	.90
Montana Center on Rural Aging Survey	Montana farmers/ranchers (mean age: 65.7) ($N = 248$)	.92
Montana Cardiac Rehabilitation Project	Rural Montana and Nevada men and women (mean age: 64) with a recent cardiac incident ($N = 286$)	.92
Women to Women Project—Cohort 1–T5	Rural middlescent women living with a chronic condition ($N = 25$)	.92
Women to Women Project—Cohort 3–T3	Rural middlescent women living with a chronic condition ($N = 27$)	.94

The current SPSS procedures that approximate Rao's factoring are maximum likelihood, and oblique rotation is direct oblimin. Using sub-sample 1 data, a 5-factor solution was first tested. Based on the magnitude of the eigenvalues, the point of discontinuity of the percentage of explained variance, and distribution of the variables within the factors, the 5-factor hypothesized

TABLE 13.2 Factor Structure and Items

Factor 1	Factor 2	Factor 3
Q-1		
Q-4		
Q-11		
Q-13		
Q-15		
	Q-2	
	Q-3	
	Q-6	
	Q-9	
	Q-12	
		Q-5
		Q-7
		Q-8
		Q-10
		Q-14

structure was not substantiated. Using the same extraction and rotation, 4-, 3-, and 2-factor structures were then examined. The 3 factors appeared to be the most suitable model and explained 46.2% of the variance. As in the earlier analyses, weak items were again noted. To identify the strongest, most parsimonious, and least redundant combination of items, the factor analysis was repeated sequentially, thus removing items that loaded heavily on 2 or more factors until a stable 3-factor solution with 15 items was identified. This model explained 54.1% of the variance, with each of the factors containing 5 items. Although items originally designed to tap the dimensions of intimacy, social integration, nurturance, worth, and assistance were represented in the reduced item model, these items did not empirically cluster as initially hypothesized. Factor 1 was composed of three of the original Intimacy items and one each of Social Integration and Worth. Factor 2 was composed of one Nurturance, one Social Integration item, and three Worth items. Factor 3 was composed of three Social Integration items and two Assistance items (Table 13.2). The alpha for the 15-item scale was .91, which was down slightly from the 25-item alpha of 0.93. The items on the PRQ appear to tap the multidimensional construct of social support, but they do not empirically arrange in the five hypothetical categories.

The intercorrelations among the three factors were: $r = .60$ between factor 1 and 2, $r = .61$ between factor 1 and 3, and $r = .70$ between factors 2 and 3. Low to moderate correlations would be anticipated if each factor contributed uniquely to the total construct. Higher correlations indicated some lack of distinctiveness of factors and redundancy in measurement. The inter-factor correlations indicated some overlapping that might be attributed to the fact that 4 items, although loading most heavily on one factor, also loaded on a second factor.

The factors were examined for internal consistency. The alpha for factor 1 was .83, factor 2 was .86, and factor 3 was .82. The inter-item correlations for factor 1 ranged from $r = .39$ to $r = .56$, for factor 2 from $r = .44$ to $r = .70$, and for factor 3 from $r = .38$ to $r = .63$, indicating that the items were correlated, as would be expected, but not with a great deal of redundancy. The factor to total correlations were $r = .81$ for factor 1, $r = .90$ for factor 2, and $r = .89$ for factor 3, indicating that each factor was highly correlated with and contributed fairly evenly to the total.

Sub-sample 2 Analysis

To explore the generalizability of the factor analysis results for sub-sample 1, analysis of sub-sample 2 was done. The process and procedures used for the analysis of sub-sample 1 were repeated. Again, the 3-factor solution appeared to be the most suitable model and explained 49.0% of the variance. The sequential factor analyses again identified a 15-item, 3-factor solution. The items loaded on the same factors as in the sub-sample 1 analysis with the exception of one item. This item loaded most heavily on factor 2 with a lighter loading on factor 3. In the sub-sample 1 analysis, this item loaded only on factor 3. The alpha for the 15-item scale was 0.90, which was down slightly from the 25-item alpha of 0.91.

The intercorrelations among the three factors were $r = .58$ between factors 1 and 2, $r = .56$ between factors 1 and 3, and $r = .69$ between factors 2 and 3. The alpha for factor 1 was .82, factor 2 was .81, and factor 3 was .79. The inter-item correlations for factor 1 ranged from $r = .35$ to $r = .63$, for factor 2 from $r = .37$ to $r = .55$, and for factor 3 from $r = .26$ to $r = .57$, indicating again that the items were correlated, but not with a great deal of redundancy. The factor to total correlations were $r = .81$ for factor 1, $r = .89$ for factor 2, and $r = .88$ for factor 3, which indicated that each factor was highly correlated with and contributed fairly evenly to the total. The results from sub-sample 2 substantiated the three-sub-scale multidimensional definition of social support. Likewise, it was demonstrated that the more parsimonious 15-item scale had similar reliability estimates for both sub-samples and did not vary dramatically from the alphas for the full 25-item scale for each sub-sample.

DESCRIPTION, ADMINISTRATION, AND SCORING

PRQ85–Part 1

The PRQ85–Part 1 was designed to estimate the number of interpersonal resources and contained 10 life situations developed to represent the domains of events for which a person might need assistance. The 10 life situations tapped the domains of (a) immediate help, (b) extended help with an ill family member, (c) relationship problems with spouse/partner or intimate other, (d) problem with a family member or friend, (e) financial problems, (f) loneliness, (g) help if sick, (h) job problems, (i) frustration with conditions of life, and (j) personal concerns. For each life situation, the respondent indicated the sources of support (e.g., no one, child, or friend). The respondent then indicated if the situation had occurred in the past 3 to 4 months and to what extent satisfaction was felt with the assistance received. Part 1 will not be included in the PRQ2000 for a variety of reasons. Because Part 1 and Part 2 can be administered independently, most researchers have not used Part 1. It significantly increased the length of the instrument and taps only assistance, rather than the multidimensional construct of social support. The intent of Part 1 was more of a heuristic device to give an estimate of the breadth and composition of the network. Those interested in network analysis are encouraged to use the stronger and more mature measures that are available. There is no single way to score Part 1, the strength of this being that investigators could use the data as best fit their particular needs. Additionally, there was no real comparability across studies. Attempts to correlate the findings of Part 1 and Part 2 were not conclusive. Thus, Part 1 will not be included as an official part of the PRQ2000. However, the PRQ85–Part 1 will be available on request and can be administered with or without the PRQ2000.*

PRQ2000

The PRQ2000 is a self-administered instrument composed of 15 items on a 7-point Likert scale that measures social support (see Appendix). The concept of social support is defined based on Weiss's (1969, 1974) model of relational functions. The item responses range from 1 (*strongly disagree*) to 7 (*strongly agree*). The 15 items are summed to calculate the total score. Possible total scores can range from 15 to 105, with higher scores indicating higher levels of perceived social support. In the developmental work, the mean scores for sub-sample 1, sub-sample 2, and several available data sets were calculated and are presented in Table 13.3.

RELIABILITY AND VALIDITY

Although the psychometric properties of the PRQ85 were demonstrated to be strong, the new PRQ2000 will need to be re-evaluated over time. As

---

*To receive the instrument, contact the author at www.montana.edu/cweinert.

TABLE 13.3 PRQ2000: Initial Mean Scores and Reliability Estimates

Study	Sample	Mean SD	Alpha
Sub-sample 1	National sample of couples (mean age: 48.4) living with multiple sclerosis (N = 449)	82.42 (14.43)	.914
Sub-sample 2	National sample of couples (mean age: 48.0) living with multiple sclerosis (N = 450)	84.72 (13.73)	.899
Women to Women Project—Out-of-State	Rural women (mean age: 50.9) living with chronic illness (N = 97)	79.72 (16.75)	.927
Montana Family Survey	Rural Montana, Wyoming, Washington, North Dakota men and women (mean age: 46.8) (N = 304)	86.24 (11.66)	.872
Montana Center on Rural Aging Survey	Montana farmers/ranchers (mean age: 65.7) (N = 248)	83.48 (13.76)	.906
Montana Family Cancer Project	Montana and Northern Wyoming persons with cancer and their caregiver (mean age: 59.2) (N = 555)	83.72 (12.93)	.904
Montana Cardiac Rehabilitation Project	Rural Montana and Nevada men and women (mean age: 64) with a recent cardiac incident (N = 286)	81.44 (14.16)	.896
Women to Women Project—T3	Rural women (mean age: 48.6) living with a chronic condition (N = 99)	79.79 (14.79)	.916

part of the developmental process discussed earlier, the new version of the Personal Resource Questionnaire was initially tested with available data sets. Reliability estimates indicated that the internal consistency remained stable and adequate, ranging from alpha = .87 to .93 (Table 13.3).

Construct validity, the extent to which a particular measure relates to other measures consistent with theoretically derived hypotheses concerning the concepts that are being measured, was evaluated for the PRQ82 (Weinert, 1987). Social support can be expected to be related to, but not the same as, mental health variables. Based on the discriminate validity principle, the PRQ ought to be correlated mid to low levels with mental health measures, thus indicating that social support is related to these constructs but is not the same. For a sample of 181 adults, the PRQ82–Part 2 was correlated with the Beck Depression Inventory (BDI; Beck,

1967) and the State-Trait Anxiety Scale (Spielberger, Gorsuch, & Lushene, 1970). Significant moderate correlations were obtained between PRQ82 and BDI ($r = -.42$) and PRQ82 and State-Trait Anxiety Scale ($r = -.39$). Norbeck and associates (Norbeck, Lindsey, & Carrieri, 1981) reported a correlation of $r = .46$ between the PRQ82 and the Profile of Mood States (POMS; McNair, 1971). The strength and direction of these correlations were consistent with the conceptualization of social support and were related to, but different from, these mental health constructs.

Construct validation was also conducted for the PRQ85. For a sample of 100 adults (mean age: 33 years), the PRQ85 was correlated with the Beck Depression Scale, the State-Trait Anxiety Scale, and the Eysenck Personality Inventory (Eysenck & Eysenck, 1968). Social support was found to be moderately associated with anxiety, depression, neuroticism, and extroversion. The correlation for the PRQ85 and depression was $r = -.42$, for anxiety $r = -.37$, for neuroticism $r = -.28$, and for extroversion $r = .32$. The direction and strength of the correlations substantiated construct validity.

To begin the process of assessing validity for the PRQ2000, available data sets, with comparable mental health measures, were examined. For the two developmental sub-samples, a depression scale, the Center for Epidemiologic Studies Depression Scale (CES-D; Devine & Orme, 1985), was available. For sub-sample 1, the correlation between the PRQ2000 and the CES-D was $r = -.51$ ($p < .001$) and for sub-sample 2 it was $r = -.44$ ($p < .001$). These sub-samples were derived from the fifth data collection point of the Family Health Study. The data from T2 were used to further the initial validity examination. For this sample of 1,199 adults living with a long-term illness, the correlation was $r = -.46$ ($p < .001$). Several additional data sets were available and appropriate for examination. First, for the Montana Family Cancer Project, a sample of 555 rural individuals with cancer and their caregivers, the correlation between the PRQ2000 and the CES-D was $r = -.44$ ($p < .001$). Second, from the Montana Family Survey, a sample of 304 rural dwellers, the correlation between the PRQ2000 and the CES-D was $r = -.25$ ($p < .001$). The third data set was from the Montana Cardiac Rehabilitation Project containing a sample of 286 rural dwellers who had experienced a cardiac incident. In this study, the Profile of Mood States (McNair, 1971) was administered, and the correlation with the PRQ2000 was $r = -.24$ ($p < .001$). Based on the divergent validity principle, measures of different constructs should have a low correlation with each other (Waltz, Strickland & Lenz, 1984). This preliminary examination gives evidence of divergent validity. As with the results from the construct validation efforts for the PRQ82 and PRQ85, these preliminary findings for the PRQ2000 again substantiated that social support is related to mental health constructs in the anticipated direction and strength.

CONCLUSIONS AND RECOMMENDATIONS

The more parsimonious PRQ2000 contains 15 items to tap the level of perceived social support and does not contain a section to estimate interpersonal resources. Results of the evaluation of the multidimensionality, using two subsamples of the same data set, did not substantiate the hypothesized five factors developed based on Weiss's (1969, 1974) five dimensions. A 3-factor structure appeared to best describe the underlying dimensions of the scale. In future studies, which have an adequate sample size, the 3-factor solution needs to be further examined. The estimates of internal consistency for the 15-item scale appeared to be as consistently strong as those for the 25-item scale. This will need to be validated each time the PRQ2000 is administered. Preliminary construct validity estimates are similar to those found for the PRQ82 and PRQ85. Extensive research, designed to evaluate the validity of the new scale, is critical. As with the previous versions of the PRQ, the scale is designed for use with English-speaking adults. The appropriateness of the use of the scale with adolescents or with non-English-speaking participants will need to be assessed.

Over the history of the Personal Resource Questionnaire, our philosophy has been that the more use the instrument got, the better. As in the past, the cost of the instrument will be kept low (copying and postage charges only). We continue to encourage researchers to reproduce as many copies as are needed and for educators to share the scale with students. Those willing to send their findings from the use of the scale will enhance our psychometric evaluation efforts. We are currently designing our Web site (www.montana.edu/cweinert) so that the PRQ2000 can be downloaded directly.

REFERENCES

Beck, A. (1967). *Depression: Causes and treatment.* Philadelphia: University of Pennsylvania Press.

Brandt, P., & Weinert, C. (1981). PRQ: A social support measure. *Nursing Research, 30,* 277–280.

Connell, K., Wayne, K., Gallant, M., & Sharpe, P. (1994). Impact of social support, social cognitive variables, and perceived threat on depression among adults with diabetes. *Health Psychology, 13,* 263–273.

Cooley, R. (1902). *Human nature and social order.* New York: Scribner.

Devine, G. & Orme, C. (1985). Center for Epidemiologic Studies Depression Scale. In D. Keyser & R. Sweetland (Eds.), *Test critiques* (Vol. 1, pp. 144–160). Kansas City, MO: Westport Publications.

Eysenck, H., & Eysenck, S. (1968). *Eysenck Personality Inventory.* San Diego, CA: Educational and Industrial Testing Services.

Faucett, J. (1994). Depression in painful chronic disorders: The role of pain and conflict about pain. *Journal of Pain and Symptom Management, 9,* 520–526.

Helgeson, V., & Cohen, S. (1996). Social support and adjustment to cancer: Reconciling descriptive, correlational, and intervention research. *Health Psychology, 15*, 135–148.

Irvine, D., Brown, B., Crooks, D., Roberts, J., & Browne, G. (1991). Psychological adjustment in women with breast cancer. *Cancer, 67*, 1097–1117.

McNair, D. (1971). *POMS manual for Profile of Mood States.* San Diego, CA: Educational and Industrial Testing Service.

Mead, G. (1934). *Mind, self and society.* Chicago: University of Chicago Press.

Moreno, J. (1934). *Who shall survive?: A new approach to the problem of human interactions.* Nervous and Mental Disease Monograph Series, (Serial No. 58). Washington, DC: Nervous and Mental Disease Publishing.

Norbeck, J., Lindsey, A., & Carrieri, V. (1981). The development of an instrument to measure social support. *Nursing Research, 30*, 264–269.

Nuckholls, K., Cassell, J., & Kaplan, G. (1972). Psychosocial assets, life crisis and prognosis of pregnancy. *American Journal of Epidemiology, 95*, 431–441.

Simmel, G. (1950). *The sociology of Georg Simmel* (K. H. Wolf, Trans). New York: Glencoe Free Press. (Original work published 1908)

Spielberger, C., Gorsuch, R., & Lushene, R. (1970). *STAI manual for the StateTrait Anxiety Questionnaire.* Palo Alto, CA: Consulting Psychologist.

Stewart, M. (1993). *Integrating social support in nursing.* Newbury Park, CA: Sage.

Thorne, S. (1993). *Negotiating health care: The social context of chronic illness.* Newbury Park, CA: Sage.

Tilden, V., & Weinert, C. (1987). Social support and the chronically ill individual. *Nursing Clinics of North America, 22*, 613–620.

Waltz, C., Strickland, O., & Lenz, E. (1984). *Measurement in nursing research.* Philadelphia: F.A. Davis.

Weinert, C. (1984). Evaluation of the PRQ: A social support measure. In K. Barnard, P. Brandt, & B. Raff (Eds.), *Social support and families of vulnerable infants* (Birth Defects, Original Article Series, 20, pp. 59–97). White Plains, NY: March of Dimes Defects Foundation.

Weinert, C. (1987). A social support measure: PRQ85. *Nursing Research, 36*, 273–277.

Weinert, C. (1988). Measuring social support: Revision and further development of the Personal Resource Questionnaire. In C. Waltz, & O. Strickland (Eds.), *Measurement of nursing outcomes* (pp. 309–327). New York: Springer Publishing Co.

Weinert, C. (2000). Social support in cyberspace. *Rehabilitation Nursing, 25*, 129–135.

Weinert, C., & Brandt, P. (1987). Measuring social support with the PRQ. *Western Journal of Nursing Research, 9*, 589–602.

Weiss, R. (1969). The fund of sociability. *TransAction, 6*(9), 36–43.

Weiss, R. (1974). The provision of social relationships. In Z. Rubin (Ed.), *Doing unto others* (pp. 17–26). Englewood Cliffs, NJ: Prentice-Hall.

Wortman, C. (1984). Social support and the cancer patient. *Cancer, 53*(Suppl., May 15), 2339–2360.

APPENDIX: PERSONAL RESOURCE QUESTIONNAIRE (PRQ2000)

Below are some statements with which some people agree and others disagree. Please read each statement and **CIRCLE** the response most appropriate for you. There is no *right* or *wrong* answer.

1 STRONGLY DISAGREE
2 DISAGREE
3 SOMEWHAT DISAGREE
4 NEUTRAL
5 SOMEWHAT AGREE
6 AGREE
7 STRONGLY AGREE

Q-1. There is someone I feel close to who makes me feel secure   1 2 3 4 5 6 7

Q-2. I belong to a group in which I feel important   1 2 3 4 5 6 7

Q-3. People let me know that I do well at my work (job, homemaking)   1 2 3 4 5 6 7

Q-4. I have enough contact with the person who makes me feel special   1 2 3 4 5 6 7

Q-5. I spend time with others who have the same interests that I do   1 2 3 4 5 6 7

Q-6. Others let me know that they enjoy working with me (job, committees, projects)   1 2 3 4 5 6 7

Q-7. There are people who are available if I need help over an extended period of time   1 2 3 4 5 6 7

Q-8. Among my group of friends we do favors for each other   1 2 3 4 5 6 7

Q-9. I have the opportunity to encourage others to develop their interests and skills   1 2 3 4 5 6 7

Q-10. I have relatives or friends who will help me out even if I can't pay them back   1 2 3 4 5 6 7

Q-11. When I am upset, there is someone I can be with who lets me be myself   1 2 3 4 5 6 7

Q-12. I know that others appreciate me as a person   1 2 3 4 5 6 7

Q-13. There is someone who loves and cares about me   1 2 3 4 5 6 7

Q-14. I have people to share social events and fun activities with   1 2 3 4 5 6 7

Q-15. I have a sense of being needed by another person   1 2 3 4 5 6 7

14

The Social Support in Chronic Illness Inventory

Gail A. Hilbert-McAllister

This chapter discusses the Social Support in Chronic Illness Inventory, a measure of the perceived satisfaction with social support received by chronically ill persons.

PURPOSE

Social support is a concept that has received much attention in the literature in recent years because of its stress buffering and its direct effects on a variety of health-related outcomes. Nurses have intuitively involved the patient's support system when planning care, realizing that family and friends are important influences. If nurses are to involve the support system more effectively for patients with chronic illness, they need to know which behaviors are supportive, in which situations, and who is best able to provide those kinds of support. However, there have been problems in designing research to provide that knowledge because of inadequate conceptualization and measurement of the support variable. This becomes increasingly important as experts in the field of social support (Gottlieb, 1985; Norbeck, 1985; Tilden, 1985; Wortman & Conway, 1985) call for clinically focused social support studies with the use of situation-specific measures. Norbeck (1985) suggested that an instrument be developed that addresses the commonalities in the demands of coping with a chronic illness. Therefore, the purpose of this chapter is to describe the Social Support in Chronic Illness Inventory, a tool for the measurement of social support related to chronic illness. The purpose of the instrument is to examine behaviors supplied by individuals experiencing a chronic illness. The instrument is designed in such a way that the respondent may give support information in relation to any individual or in relation to a specific group of individuals such as friends or fellow workers.

CONCEPTUAL BASIS OF THE SOCIAL SUPPORT IN CHRONIC ILLNESS INVENTORY

The theoretical framework on which the development of the Social Support in Chronic Illness Inventory (SSCII) was based is twofold: the concept of the convoy (Kahn, 1979; Kahn & Quinn, 1976) and a model of stress, coping, and health (Hogue, 1977; Kahn, 1979).

Kahn and Quinn (1976) define the convoy as a metaphorical term implying "that each person can be thought of as moving through life surrounded by a set of significant other people to whom that person is related by giving or receiving of social support" (p. 10). This concept bears similarity to role set but differs in two important ways. First, it is defined by the giving and receiving of social support rather than by a person's position in a formal organization. Second, and perhaps more important, the convoy implies movement, whereas a role is more static.

The concept of the convoy was chosen for the development of the present instrument because it carries with it the notions of person–environment interaction and change over time, both important in the conceptualization of nursing. The convoy implies that support needs change with time and are dependent on the characteristics of the person and the environment. This is seen to be congruent with an instrument that measures social support in chronic illness as supplied by individuals who are most important to the recipient at that point in his or her life. It is expected that the amount and kinds of support needed will vary with characteristics of the individual and characteristics of the illness, but that patterns will emerge that will be useful to nurses who are assessing social support resources of clients and planning interventions to increase support when deficiencies are noted.

The model of stress, coping, and health is a combination of those used by Kahn and Quinn (1976) and Hogue (1977). The former focuses on the social support convoy and the latter on the more specific steps of the stress-coping model.

In this model, personal and social resources are considered together as coping resources, both of which determine whether or not potentially threatening situations lead to responses supportive of health or illness. "Coping resources may influence whether or not situations are perceived as threatening to a given person; they may allow persons who perceive threat to deal creatively with the threat, and/or they may influence the impact of health changes on the individual" (Hogue, 1977, p. 66). Kahn (1979) sees the research utility of the convoy in the specification and measurement of properties of the convoy as a whole, as well as properties of the separate dyadic links between the focal person and each of the convoy members.

The theoretical definition used in the development of the SSCII is based on Barrera and Ainlay's (1983) review of the social support literature. Social support is defined as a diversity of natural helping behaviors of which individuals are recipients in social interactions: tangible aid (material aid and behavioral assistance), intimate interaction, guidance, feedback, and positive social interaction. This definition is congruent with the theoretical framework and was chosen because (1) it is based on a review of the extant social support literature, (2) it subsumes most other categories of support that have been deductively derived, and (3) it is compatible with Gottlieb's (1978) categories of natural helping behaviors, which were inductively derived.

The SSCII is used for support in relation to chronic illness, such as hypertension, diabetes, cardiac disease, and end-stage renal disease. All of these diagnoses carry with them the necessity for long-term lifestyle adjustments, especially in the areas of activity, diet, and medication. As several authors have noted (Cohen & Syme, 1985; Dimond, 1985), it is important to examine the need for support longitudinally, an approach that is congruent with the theoretical framework of the convoy.

The concept of the convoy does not include the dimension of organized support. Kahn and Quinn (1976) define convoys as "natural helping groups" (p. 4). The items that were developed for the SSCII cover the broad range of supportive behaviors, many of which are found primarily in natural supportive relationships, such as expressions of affection and spending time together in social interaction. Therefore, the questionnaire has less utility for assessing supportive functions of organized relationships.

The SSCII is designed in such a way that responses may be subjective or objective, in the sense that the items may be completed by either the recipient or the provider of the support in relation to the frequency with which the behaviors are supplied. Respondents may also be asked to indicate the quality of the support received by indicating their degree of satisfaction with each behavior, as indicated in the directions on the questionnaire (see Appendix).

PROCEDURES FOR DEVELOPMENT

The literature was reviewed to locate social support measures that focus on specific behaviors of supportive individuals rather than on the network or global measures of satisfaction with received support. Four scales were located that contained specific behaviors contributing to social support for individuals in a variety of situations: the Inventory of Socially Supportive Behaviors (ISSB; Barrera & Ainlay, 1983), Social Support Items (SSI; Lin, Dean, & Ensel, 1981), the Social Support Questionnaire (SSQ; Sarason, Levine, Basham, & Sarason, 1983), and the Perceived Support for Friends/Family (PSS-Fr, PSS-Fa; Procidano & Heller, 1983). Additionally, two instruments were located that were appropriate for health-related situations: the Support Behaviors Inventory (SBI; Brown, 1986) and the Spouse Support Questionnaire (SSQ; Hilbert, 1983). However, none of these instruments measure all aspects of social support in relation to chronic illness.

Forty-five items were developed for the SSCII based on the literature, previously developed questionnaires (including the ISSB, SSQ-Hilbert, SSI, PSS-Fr, PSS-Fa, and SSQ), and interviews with myocardial infarction (MI) patients (Hilbert, 1983). Sixty-four percent of the items are from the Spouse Support Questionnaire (Hilbert, 1983). The derivation and content mapping of items on the SSCII can be found in Hilbert (1990).

A decision was made to measure perceived satisfaction with each of the supportive behaviors. The literature review indicated conflicting opinions about whether quality is a more significant dimension than quantity. However, previous research with MI patients indicated that satisfaction with support appeared to be more important than the number of times a behavior occurred (Hilbert, 1983).

DESCRIPTION

The Social Support in Chronic Illness Inventory consists of 38 Likert-scale items. The items were placed on a 6-point Likert scale ranging from *dissatisfied* to *very satisfied*. General support items were included for all categories of Barrera and Ainlay's (1983) social support. Specific items were included for guidance and feedback. Material aid and behavioral assistance were combined to form a Tangible Assistance subscale, based on the report of a factor analysis that showed those items loading together (Barrera & Ainlay, 1983) and in order to have each subscale contain at least four items. Items 1 to 10 form the Intimate Interaction subscale; 11–17 and 30–36, the Guidance subscale; 18–20, 37, and 38, the Feedback subscale; 21–24, the Tangible Assistance subscale; and 25–29, the Positive Social Interaction subscale.

ADMINISTRATION AND SCORING

Using a paper-and-pencil format, subjects are instructed to identify the one person who is most important to them at the present time. They are asked to note how satisfied they are with the helping behaviors of that person toward them in the past month. Scores for each of the 38 items are summed, with a possible range of 38 to 228. The higher the score, the greater the degree of satisfaction with the support supplied by the person named as most important to the subject. Time required for completing the questionnaire is 10 to 15 minutes

RELIABILITY AND VALIDITY EVIDENCE

Two experts in the area of social support assessed the posteriori content validity of the SSCII. These experts rated each of the 45 original items for relevancy to the purpose of the instrument on a 4-point scale. The 38 items with 100% agreement as very relevant or quite relevant were retained. The result was 29 general-support items and 9 chronic illness–specific items.

Sample

A sample of 190 chronically ill persons was recruited from a variety of sites, including diabetic education centers, blood pressure screenings, health fairs, hemodialysis clinics, and cardiac rehabilitation centers. Chronic illness was defined as an altered health state that will not be cured by a simple surgical procedure or a short course of therapy (Miller, 1983). Delimitations included no concurrent acute illness and a diagnosis of at least one of the following: hypertension, diabetes, cardiac disease, or end-stage renal disease. Informed consent was obtained.

A little more than half (54%) of the sample were females. Average age was 56 years; average education was 13 years. The majority of subjects were White (76%), with 19% Black, 4% American Indian, and 1% Hispanic. Two thirds were married, and 14% were widowed. Forty-nine percent had diabetes; 35%, heart disease; 66%, hypertension; and 35%, end-stage renal disease. This adds up to over 100% because many had more than one diagnosis. Average time since diagnosis was as follows: diabetes, 12 years; heart disease, 7 years; hypertension, 12 years; and end-stage renal disease, 2.7 years. Fifty-eight percent of respondents named the spouse as the most supportive person, with daughter named in second place in 13% of responses.

Distribution of Scores

The range of scores on the SSCII for this sample was 74 to 228, with 36 subjects (19% of the sample) having the maximum score of 228. The mean was 195, and the standard deviation was 33.9.

Reliability

Coefficient alpha for the total scale was .98. Reliability coefficients for the subscales ranged from .84 to .94, as shown in Table 14.1. The individual

TABLE 14.1 Reliabilities and Intercorrelations of Support Subscales

	Intimate interaction	Guidance	Feedback	Tangible aid	Positive social interaction
Intimate interaction	[.95]	.80	.75	.56	.78
Guidance	[.95]	.87	.69	.70	
Feedback	[.93]	.69	.81		
Tangible aid	[.84]	.67			
Positive social interaction	[.92]				

Note: Numbers in brackets are internal consistency reliability coefficients.

items demonstrated item-to-total correlations ranging from .56 to .87. Correlations between subscales ranged from .56 to .87.

Validity Assessment Using Factor Analysis

A principal-component factor analysis without iteration (Nie, Hull, Jenkins, Steinbrenner, & Bent, 1970) was done as an assessment of construct validity. There was a subject-to-item ratio of 5 to 1 for the factor analysis procedure. Inspection of the eigenvalues of the factors, the points of discontinuity of the percentage of explained variance, and the distribution of the variables within the factors did not substantiate the five theorized factors. Using the criteria of including variables that loaded at .40 or higher and also showed at least .15 difference from high loadings on other factors, three factors were identified.

Factor 1 clearly included all of the items that were theorized to measure intimate interaction. One additional variable loaded on that factor: "shared an interest" (positive social interaction). Factor 2 included six of the seven items in the specific guidance subscale. Factor 3 included two of the five items from the Positive Social Interaction Subscale. All of the Positive Social Interaction items also loaded at .40 or above on factor 1.

Eigenvalues for factors 1, 2, and 3 were 21.48, 3.23, and 1.58, respectively. The decrease in eigenvalues after factor 1 indicated one main factor and two less important factors. Although this may have been an indication that social support in chronic illness is a unidimensional concept, it may also have been an artifact of the principal-component factor analysis, which searches for the most economical set of relationships that are expressed in the first factor.

To further test the one-factor solution, a Rao canonical factor analysis was done (Nie et al., 1970). This procedure seeks a specified number of factors to account for the observed correlation matrix. The results confirmed the one main factor explanation in that the first factor accounted for 74.4% of the variance.

CONCLUSIONS AND RECOMMENDATIONS

The high reliability for the total scale, the correlations among subscales, and the results of the factor analyses suggest that social support in chronic illness is a unidimensional concept. However, the factors that did emerge are consistent with three of the five categories of support that were theorized. Reports in the literature on unidimensionality versus multidimensionality of support are conflicting. Although Barrera and Ainlay (1983) reported four categories of supportive behavior based on their factor analysis of the ISSB, Stokes and Wilson (1984) found the ISSB to be a global measure of support. Brown (1986) reported a dominant construct of social support during pregnancy that organized at the broad level. In the study of MI patients, Hilbert (1983) found two clearly delineated categories of support that were similar to intimate interaction and directive guidance.

The variations in the findings may have been caused by the homogeneous versus heterogeneous nature of the samples. It may be that several dimensions of support emerge in clearly delimited samples experiencing similar stresses. For the present study, it would appear that for those with chronic illness, emotional support and specific guidance are important factors in their perceptions of social support, with emotional support emerging as the primary factor.

The majority of subjects in the present sample were beyond the period of initial adjustment to the demands of their illness. For them, generalized emotional support would assume more importance than specific guidance. The specific guidance factor was second in importance and clearly less significant. The results of the factor analysis might be different for those who are newly diagnosed. Those individuals would need more guidance in carrying out the specific demands of the regimens. It is recommended that further validation studies be conducted, using approaches such as experimental manipulation and hypothesis testing.

ACKNOWLEDGMENT

This research was supported by a grant from the Xi chapter of Sigma Theta Tau.

REFERENCES

Barrera, M., & Ainlay, S. L. (1983). The structure of social support: A conceptual and empirical analysis. *Journal of Community Psychology, 11,* 133–143.
Brown, M. A. (1986). Social support during pregnancy: A unidimensional or multidimensional construct? *Nursing Research, 35,* 4–9.

Cohen, S., & Syme, S. L. (1985). Issues in the study and application of social support. In S. Cohen & S.L. Syme (Eds.), *Social support and health* (pp. 3–22). Orlando, FL: Academic Press.

Dimond, M. (1985). A review and critique of the concepts of social support. In R. A. O'Brien (Coordinator), *Social support health: New directions for theory development and research.* Symposium conducted at the University of Rochester (pp. 1–32), Rochester, NY.

Gottlieb, B. H. (1978). The development and application of a classification scheme of informal helping behaviors. *Canadian. Journal of Behavioral Science, 10,* 105–115.

Gottlieb, B. H. (1985). Marshaling and augmenting social support for medical patients and their families. *Social support and health: New directions for theory development and research.* (pp. 107–148). Symposium conducted at the University of Rochester, Rochester, NY.

Hilbert, G. A. (1983). *The relationship between spouse support and compliance of myocardial infarction patients.* Unpublished doctoral dissertation, University of Pennsylvania, Philadelphia.

Hilbert, G. A. (1990). Measuring social support in chronic illness. In O. L. Strickland & C. F. Waltz, *Measurement of nursing outcomes: Measuring client self-care and coping skills* (Vol. 4, pp. 79–95). New York: Springer.

Hogue, D. D. (1977). Support systems for health promotion. In J. E. Hall & B. R. Weaver (Eds.), *Distributive nursing practice: A systems approach for community health* (pp. 65–79). Philadelphia: J. B. Lippincott.

Kahn, R. L. (1979). Aging and social support. In M. W. Riley (Ed.), *Aging from birth to death: Interdisciplinary perspectives* (pp. 77–91). Boulder, CO: Westview.

Kahn, R. L., & Quinn, R. P. (1976). *Mental health, social support and metropolitan problems.* Unpublished manuscript, Institute for Social Research, University of Michigan, Ann Arbor.

Lin, N., Dean, A., & Ensel, W. M. (1981). Social support scales: A methodological note *Schizophrenia Bulletin, 7,* 73–89.

Miller, J. F. (1983). *Coping with chronic illness: Overcoming powerlessness.* Philadelphia: F. A. Davis.

Nie, N. H., Hull, C. H., Jenkins, J. G., Steinbrenner, K., & Bent, D. J. (1970). *Statistical package for the social sciences.* New York: McGraw-Hill.

Norbeck, J. S. (1985). Measurement of social support: Recent strategies and continuing issues. In *Social support and health: New directions for theory development and research.* (pp. 73–106), Symposium conducted at the University of Rochester, Rochester, NY.

Procidano, M. E., & Heller, K. (1983). Measures of perceived social support from friends and family: Three validation studies. *American Journal of Community Psychology, 11,* 1–24.

Sarason, I. G., Levine, H. M., Basham, R. B., & Sarason, B. R. (1983). Assessing social support: The Social Support Questionnaire. *Journal of Personality and Social Psychology, 44,* 127–139.

Stokes, J., & Wilson, D. G. (1984). Inventory of socially supportive behaviors: Dimensionality, prediction, and gender differences. *American Journal of Community Psychology, 2,* 53–64.

Tilden, V. (1985). Issues of conceptualization and measurement of social support in the construction of nursing theory. *Research in Nursing and Health, 8,* 199–206.

Wortman, C. B., & Conway, T. L. (1985). The role of social support in adaptation and recovery from physical illness. In S. Cohen & S. L. Syme (Eds.), *Social support and health* (pp. 281–302). Orlando, FL: Academic Press.

APPENDIX: SOCIAL SUPPORT IN CHRONIC ILLNESS INVENTORY

Directions

This section refers to the person whom you named as most important to you in terms of being helpful on a day-to-day basis. In the past month, how satisfied were you with the helping behaviors of that person toward you? Indicate your degree of satisfaction with each behavior listed below by circling the number that applies to you. The number 1 indicates dissatisfaction. The number 6 indicates that you are very satisfied.

HOW SATISFIED ARE YOU WITH
THE AMOUNT THE PERSON YOU
NAMED DOES THIS FOR YOU?

1 = Dissatisfied
2 = Somewhat dissatisfied
3 = Partly satisfied
4 = Somewhat satisfied
5 = Satisfied
6 = Very satisfied

1. Told me that I am OK just the way I am.	1 2 3 4 5 6
2. Comforted me by showing some physical affection.	1 2 3 4 5 6
3. Let me know that (s)he can be counted on if I need help.	1 2 3 4 5 6
4. Expressed interest and concern in my well-being.	1 2 3 4 5 6
5. Told me that (s)he feels very close to me.	1 2 3 4 5 6
6. Was available to listen when I wanted to talk.	1 2 3 4 5 6
7. Enjoyed hearing about what I think.	1 2 3 4 5 6
8. Consoled me when I was upset.	1 2 3 4 5 6
9. Allowed me to come to him/her when I was feeling down.	1 2 3 4 5 6
10. Accepted me totally, including my worst and best parts.	1 2 3 4 5 6
11. Made it clear what was expected of me.	1 2 3 4 5 6
12. Gave me some information on how to do something.	1 2 3 4 5 6
13. Gave me some information to help me understand a situation I was in.	1 2 3 4 5 6
14. Told me who I should see for assistance	1 2 3 4 5 6
15. Told me what to expect in a situation that was about to happen.	1 2 3 4 5 6
16. Taught me how to do something.	1 2 3 4 5 6

	1 = Dissatisfied	2 = Somewhat dissatisfied	3 = Partly satisfied	4 = Somewhat satisfied	5 = Satisfied	6 = Very satisfied
17. Talked with me about a problem in order to help solve it.	1	2	3	4	5	6
18. Checked back with me to see if I had followed the advice I was given.	1	2	3	4	5	6
19. Helped me understand why I didn't do something well.	1	2	3	4	5	6
20. Gave me feedback on how I was doing without saying it was good or bad.	1	2	3	4	5	6
21. Contributed to my income or gave me money.	1	2	3	4	5	6
22. Gave me a gift.	1	2	3	4	5	6
23. Did a task that is usually done by me.	1	2	3	4	5	6
24. Provided transportation for me.	1	2	3	4	5	6
25. Did some activity together to help me get my mind off of things.	1	2	3	4	5	6
26. Talked with me about some interests of mine.	1	2	3	4	5	6
27. Joked or kidded to try to cheer me up.	1	2	3	4	5	6
28. Shared an interest.	1	2	3	4	5	6
29. Could count on her/him to distract me form worries.	1	2	3	4	5	6
30. Shared information with me about recommendations that were made by the health team.	1	2	3	4	5	6
31. Helped me to understand about my disease.	1	2	3	4	5	6
32. Told me whom I should see for assistance when I had problems with the health team recommendations.	1	2	3	4	5	6
33. Told me how useful the health team recommendations were in preventing complications.	1	2	3	4	5	6
34. Taught me how to carry out the health team recommendations.	1	2	3	4	5	6
35. Talked with me about problems I was having with the health team recommendations.	1	2	3	4	5	6
36. Encouraged me to take proper care of myself.	1	2	3	4	5	6
37. Checked back to see if I had carried out recommendations I consider important.	1	2	3	4	5	6
38. Commented favorably when (s)he noticed me doing something that the health team recommended.	1	2	3	4	5	6

15

The Caring Ability Inventory

Ngozi O. Nkongho

This chapter discusses the Caring Ability Inventory, a tool that measures one's ability to care when involved in a relationship with others.

PURPOSE

It is generally recognized that people feel and behave differently in different relationships with others. One possible explanation for this difference relates to the amount of caring present and felt by those involved. Not only do we need to measure the ability of health care providers to care, but also the ability of family members to care for one another. This measure may be used to assess the caring ability of abusive parents, clients who are unable to maintain relationships and nurses and other health care providers who work with patients. To increase our understanding of human relationships, it is essential that people's caring ability be analyzed and quantified. With this knowledge, it is possible to identify areas of weakness and strength in a person's ability to care. Intervention strategies can be planned based on these findings.

The purpose of the Caring Ability Inventory (CAI) is to quantify a person's degree of caring ability relative to others. Specifically, the purpose of CAI is to measure the degree of a person's ability to care for others.

CONCEPTUAL BASIS OF THE CARING ABILITY INVENTORY

The conceptual framework for the CAI was derived from the literature on caring. Four theoretical assumptions were identified. Specifically, these were (1) caring is multidimensional, with cognitive and attitudinal components; (2) the potential to care is present in all individuals; (3) caring can be learned; and (4) caring is quantifiable.

184

The CAI is based on Mayeroff's (1971) discussion of caring. He defines caring as "helping another grow and actualize himself, . . . a process, a way of relating to someone that involves development" (p. 1). He identified eight indicators of caring: knowing, alternating rhythm, patience, honesty, trust, humility, hope, and courage.

Knowing involves an awareness of the other as separate, with unique needs. It implies understanding who the person cared for is, his or her needs, strengths, and weaknesses, and what enhances his or her well-being. Knowing can be explicit or implicit, direct or indirect; it includes both general and specific knowledge of the person cared for. An important aspect of knowing is knowing one's own strengths and limitations.

Alternating rhythms refers to fluctuations in the scope of caring. At times, caring involves doing for the other, and at times it may involve doing nothing. The caregiver needs to be aware of when doing and not doing represent caring. Alternating rhythm provides a basis for identifying patterns of caring. Patterns make it possible to learn from past experience what behaviors were helpful or not helpful and to modify one's actions to facilitate growth.

Patience is essential in caring because it allows time and room for self-expression and exploration. Being patient includes being tolerant of some degree of confusion and disorganization, which characterizes growth for self and others.

Honesty involves seeing others as they are instead of as the caregiver wishes them to be. The changing needs of the individual over time are visible when that person is seen as he or she is at a given time. Honesty in caring also implies being genuine or real to oneself. When one is genuine, there is congruence between what is said, what is felt, and what is done. When honesty is present, the caregiver is available and open to the other, and energy is not wasted on pretending to be what one is not.

Trust is present in caring as it allows others to grow in their own time and their own way. Trust involves having confidence in one's abilities and in the other person's abilities as well. A trusting relationship encourages and fosters independence.

Humility involves continuous learning about the other and is never completed. Different people can care for others without any particular kind of caring being more important than another. With humility, there is genuineness without the need to pretend what one is not or to conceal aspects of self. Without pretense, one can be seen truly, as a person with both strengths and limitations.

Hope is present in caring and is associated with the anticipation of growth with caring. With hope in caring, the present becomes alive and significant as the possibilities to be realized in the future are recognized.

Courage is present in caring when the direction of growth and its outcome are largely unknown. The courage to care is gained from past experience and by being sensitive and open to the needs of the present.

PROCEDURES FOR DEVELOPMENT

The work of Mayeroff (1971), in which the eight critical elements of caring were identified (knowing, alternating rhythm, patience, honesty, trust, humility, hope, and courage), provided the theoretical framework for formulating the CAI. Items were derived in two ways. First, from the review of the literature on caring and related concepts, 61 items were constructed. The second method involved interviewing 15 consenting adults on their thoughts on caring, using 10 open-ended questions, which generated specific characteristics of caring . From these interviews, 19 additional items were derived. A total of 80 items were constructed: 34 positive statements and 46 negatively worded statements. The initial inventory consisted of 80 items using a 7-point Likert scale.

The responses of 543 respondents to the original CAI items were subjected to a principal-axis factor analysis. On the basis of the screen test, as well as the interpretability of factors, it was decided that a 3-factor analysis was appropriate for these data. Both orthogonal and oblique solutions were conducted. The correlations among factors were so low in the oblique solution that an orthogonal solution was used. Items that loaded on factor 1 appeared to deal with understanding of self and others. This factor was therefore named Knowing because it approximates Mayeroff's original description of the element. Factor 2 seemed to tap ability to deal with the unknown and is named Courage. Factor 3 included items characterized by toleration and persistence and was therefore named Patience. Items were chosen for inclusion in the final three subscales only if they loaded above .30 on a given factor and did not load at the .30 level on the other factors.

DESCRIPTION

The CAI is a Likert-scale instrument with 37 items. The Likert scale is a 7-point scale ranging from 1 to 7. It has three subscales: Knowing, Courage, and Patience. The Knowing subscale consists of 14 items, Courage consists of 13 items, and Patience has 10 items. So the total CAI consists of 37 items (see CAI in Appendix). Intercorrelation of the subscales is moderate in size and reflects separate domains within the overall concept of caring. The intercorrelation of the Courage and Knowing scales was .42, for the Courage and Patience scales .19, and the Patience and Knowing scales .35.

ADMINISTRATION AND SCORING

The CAI is self-administered and requires no instructions beyond that indicated at the beginning of the inventory. The Likert-type responses range from 1 to 7, with higher scores indicating greater degree of caring for a positively phrased item. For negatively worded items, the scoring is reversed. Item responses are then summed for each subscale, yielding a total score for each subscale. Because the Knowing subscale has 14 items, the possible range of scores is from 14 to 98. The Courage subscale has 13 items, with a possible range of scores from 13 to 91. The Patience subscale has 10 items; its scores can range from 10 to 70.). The total caring ability score is a composite of the three subscales (see "Scoring Information") for items in each subscale, items to be reverse scored, and norms for nurses and college female and male students.

RELIABILITY AND VALIDITY EVIDENCE

Several studies have been conducted that provide evidence for the reliability and validity of the CAI. These studies, sample characteristics, and specific reliability and validity evidence are presented in Table 15.1.

SCORING INFORMATION

Items to be summed for each subscale:
1. Knowing: 2, 3, 6, 7, 9, 19, 22, 26, 30, 31, 33, 34, 35, 36
2. Courage: 4, 8, 11, 12, 13, 14, 15, 16, 23, 25, 28, 29, 32
3. Patience: 1, 5, 10, 17, 18, 20, 21, 24, 27, 37
4. Items to be reverse-scored: 4, 8, 11, 12, 13, 14, 15, 16, 23, 25, 28, 29, 32

Description of the Norming Procedure

The nurse group comprised 75 practicing nurses attending a national conference. Participants came from all areas of the counhy. To determine ranges for low-, medium-, and high-norm scores, 0.5 standard deviation on either side of the mean was considered to be in the middle range of scores. Scores above this were considered high, and scores below this were considered low. See Table 15.2 for low, medium, and high norms for the nurse group.

The college students group consisted of 424 females and 103 males attending a large university in metropolitan New York. The students represented a wide variety of ability, ethnic, and socioeconomic groups. Low, medium, and high groups were determined in the same way as noted above. See Table 15.3 for low, medium, and high norms for female and male college students.

TABLE 15.1 Studies Supporting the Reliability and Validity of the Caring Ability Inventory (CAI)

Study citation	Sample and characteristics	Reliability evidence	Validity evidence
Nkongho (1990)	The sample consisted of two groups: (1) 462 college students from varied majors, and (2) 75 nurses attending a national professional conference. Of the 537 respondents, 20% were male and 80% were female. Most of the sample (61%) was under the age of 33 years.	*Internal consistency:* Total CAI = .84 Subscales: Knowing = .79 Courage = .75 Patience = .71 *Test-retest:* Conducted with 38 respondents on 2 occasions, 2 weeks apart. Total CAI = .75 Subscales: Knowing = .80 Courage = .64 Patience = .73	*Content validity:* A priori content validity was supported by the fact that items were developed based on the literature and critical elements of caring identified by Mayeroff (1971). A content validity index of .80 resulted from ratings of two experts. *Construct validity:* Results from t-test analysis supported the hypothesis that practicing nurses would score higher on caring than college students for the total CAI (t = 7.06; p<.001); and each of the subscales, i. e., knowing (t = 7.95; p < .001), courage (t = 3.43; p < .001), and patience (t = 5.16; p<.001). The hypothesis that females would score higher on the CAI than males was supported (t = 5.22; p<.001). The hypothesis that there would be a positive

TABLE 15.1 (*continued*)

Study citation	Sample and characteristics	Reliability evidence	Validity evidence
Nkongho (1990) (*continued*)			relationship between self-concept scores and scores on the CAI was also supported ($r = .53$; $p < .001$). *Factor analysis:* Results indicated the presence of three factors that were compatible with the conceptual basis of the CAI.
Simmons & Cavanaugh (1996)	A national sample of 350 female senior students in U.S. baccalaureate nursing programs was randomly selected from members of the National Student Nurse Association. Median age was 23 ($M = 26.5$, $SD = 7.0$). Almost 90% were white. About 41% reported in-come levels below $20,000, 14% above $60,000.	*Internal consistency:* Cronbach's alpha for total CAI = .79.	*Construct validity:* Supported by the hypothesized relation between CAI score and perception of caring within nursing school climate (as assessed by Part A of the Charles F. Kettering Ltd. School Climate Profile). The correlation between CAI and CFK Profile scores was .16 ($p < .01$).
Cavanaugh & Simmons (1997) (*continued*)	A national sample of 495 female students (the 350 senior students in the	*Internal consistency:* Cronbach's alpha for total CAI = .79.	*Construct validity:* The correlation between total CAI score and overall

TABLE 15.1 (*continued*)

Study citation	Sample and characteristics	Reliability evidence	Validity evidence
Cavanaugh & Simmons (1997) (*continued*)	Simmons & Cavanaugh, 1996, study, along with 145 juniors) in U.S. baccalaureate nursing programs was randomly selected from members of the National Student Nurse Association. Median age was 24 ($M = 27.1$, $SD = 7.3$). About 88% were White. About 43% reported income levels below $20,000, 14% above $60,000.		nursing school climate was .24 ($p < .001$). The dimensions of school climate (Respect, Trust, Morale, Caring) that correlated most strongly with the CAI subscales were Caring; $r = .17$, .22, .17 with Patience, Knowing, and Courage, respectively ($p < .001$). Further evidence of construct validity: The total CAI mean of 208 for the nursing students was higher than the mean of 196 reported for 462 college students with varied majors by Nkongho (1990), but lower than the mean of 212 reported for 75 nurses in that study.
Simmons & Cavanaugh (2000)	In the second phase of a longitudinal study, 189 of the 495 nursing students included in the Cavanaugh and Simmons 1997 study,	*Internal consistency:* Cronbach's alpha for total CAI = .83. Evidence of the stability of CAI scores was found in the	*Construct validity:* A paired *t*-test indicated that, as hypothesized, CAI total scores were higher for graduates than for students

TABLE 15.1 *(continued)*

Study citation	Sample and characteristics	Reliability evidence	Validity evidence
Simmons & Cavanaugh (2000) *(continued)*	who had obtained their nursing degree and entered nursing practice, responded to a follow-up survey 3 years later. Almost 97% reported passing the national nursing licensing exam with more than 90% passing on the first attempt. Median age was 26 ($M = 30.3$, $SD = 7.5$). About 93% were White. About 6% reported income levels below $20,000, 4% above $60,000.	.59 correlation ($p < .001$) between student and follow-up graduate CAI scores.	($p < .001$). This cannot be attributed to maturation, as age was not found to be related to CAI in this group. Additional confirmation of construct validity: the correlation between CAI score and perception of nursing school climate was .17 ($p < .05$).
Baird (1996)	The sample consisted of 286 nursing students (58 males and 228 females) and 267 dental hygiene students (5 males and 262 females) in associate degree programs at four northeastern community colleges. The mean age of the nursing students was 30.4 ($SD = 7.8$); the mean age of the dental hygiene students was 25.8 ($SD = 6.7$).	*Internal consistency:* Cronbach's alpha for total CAI = .81 for nursing students, = .79 for dental hygiene students.	*Construct validity:* A comparison of nursing and dental hygiene student scores on the CAI provided evidence for construct validity. As hypothesized, the nursing students' mean (209.8) was higher ($p < .01$) than that of the dental hygiene students (205.5). In addition, CAI scores were correlated with scores on the Inventory of Socially Supportive Behaviors, $r = .24$, p < .001.

TABLE 15.1 (*continued*)

Study citation	Sample and characteristics	Reliability evidence	Validity evidence
Davenport (1999)	Of the 76 sophomore students at a Texas university who participated in the study, half were nursing majors and half were nonnursing majors. There were 29 males and 47 females. Median age was 22 (*M* = 25.6, *SD* = 8.5).	*Internal consistency:* Cronbach's alpha for total CAI = .84.	*Construct validity:* Evidence of construct validity was provided by the results of a *t*-test comparing non-nursing majors' and nursing majors' total CAI scores. Confirming one of the study's hypotheses, the nursing majors' mean (212.4) was found to be higher than that of the nonnursing majors (198.2), *p* < .001. Additional support for construct validity was the finding that the total CAI mean of the female nursing students (214.5) was higher than that of the male nursing students (202.9), *p* < .05.
Higgins (1993)	The sample comprised 39 male and 47 female Air Force mental health nurses. About 90% of them held ranks of captain or above.	*Internal consistency:* Cronbach's alpha for total CAI = .87.	*Construct validity:* Total CAI scores were positively related to a number of variables in this study, providing evidence for

TABLE 15.1 *(continued)*

Study citation	Sample and characteristics	Reliability evidence	Validity evidence
Higgins (1993) *(continued)*	The median age was 36. The median number of years of experience as a registered nurse was 13.		construct validity. CAI scores were correlated with years of registered nurse experience, ($r = .20$, $p < .05$), scores on the Nurses' Attitudes Toward Mental Illness Scale ($r = .31$, $p < .01$), and scores on the Power in Knowing Participation in Change Tool ($r = .55$, $p < .01$).
Nkongho (1998)	The sample was composed of 15 male and 94 female undergraduates attending a large urban university. Median age was 25 ($M = 27.5$, $SD = 7.1$). Approximately 42% identified themselves as lower middle class, 46% as middle class.	*Internal consistency:* Cronbach's alphas for total CAI = .83 *Subscales* Patience = .67 Knowing = .80 Courage = .69	*Construct validity:* As hypothesized, a relationship was found between ego development levels and CAI scores. Spearman correlation coefficients between scores on the Washington University Sentence Completion Test and the CAI were: Patience = .18 $p < .05$ Knowing = .17 $p < .05$ Courage = .29 $p < .001$ Total CAI = .28 $p < .01$

TABLE 15.2 Low, Medium, High Norms for the CAI and Its Subscales for Nurses

Subscale	Low	Medium	High
Knowing	Below 76.4	76.4—84.0	Above 84.0
Courage	Below 62.5	62.5—74.0	Above 74.0
Patience	Below 61.0	61.0—65.2	Above 65.2
Total CAI	Below 203.1	203.1—220.3	Above 220.3

CONCLUSIONS AND RECOMMENDATIONS

If the ability to care is necessary for human survival, it is important to assess the degree to which this ability is present for people in general and to identify situations under which their ability to care changes. Therefore, an instrument that measures caring ability is required. The CAI was designed to meet this need.

The CAI consists of 37 items representing 3 of the elements cited by Mayeroff (1971): Knowing, Courage, and Patience. Reliabilities for the subscales have been assessed in multiple studies using several approaches. Findings indicate that the CAI is a reliable measure of caring.

Assessment of content validity yielded a content validity index of .80. Construct validity has been estimated by discrimination between students and nurses and between females and males. Construct validity has also been supported through factor analysis and multiple studies using hypothesis testing with results consistent with theory and the literature.

The development of the CAI has many implications for nursing and other professions. The ability to care is multidimensional, with cognitive and affective domains. The CAI can be used to identify persons who are high or low on these dimensions. Individuals who are high may serve as models or mentors for those who are low on caring. The ability to care is more important in some situations and in some professions than in others. Therefore, the CAI may be used in counseling and vocational guidance.

In the care of the aged parent, a family member who is high in caring may be encouraged to assume the care of the parent, rather than a person who is less caring. The CAI may be administered at specific intervals to determine if and when changes occur. Changes in CAI scores may be an early indication of stress or burden in this relationship.

The CAI has potential implications for education. Can the dimensions of the CAI be taught? What teaching methods are appropriate? Are the dimensions of caring included as learning objectives? The CAI can be administered to new students and at each level to determine their mastery of caring constructs as students advance in their studies. In addition, the CAI can be used as a prepost measure for assessing the success of new programs or courses designed to foster caring behaviors.

TABLE 15.3 Low, Medium, High Norms for the CAI and Its Subscales for Female and Male College Students

Subscale	Females ($n = 424$)			Males ($n = 103$)		
	Low	Medium	High	Low	Medium	High
Knowing	< 68.8	68.8–79.5	> 79.5	< 64.6	64.6–75.1	> 75.11
Courage	< 62.14	62.14–73.06	> 73.06	< 54.41	54.41–66.56	> 66.56
Patience	< 58.05	58.05–64.35	> 64.35	< 53.4	53.4–62.4	> 62.4
Total CAI	< 190.29	190.29–211.12	> 211.12	< 178.00	178.00–199.36	> 199.36

REFERENCES

Baird, K. S. (1996). A comparative study of differences in caring ability and the role of social support in associate degree nursing and dental hygiene students. *Dissertation Abstracts International, 57*(7), 4292B. (UMI No. AAD 96-35950)

Cavanaugh, S., & Simmons, P. (1997). Evaluation of a school climate instrument for assessing affective objectives in health professional education. *Evaluation and the Health Professions, 20,* 455–478.

Davenport, D. (1999). *Gender differences in caring abilities among baccalaureate nursing and non-nursing students.* Unpublished manuscript.

Higgins, M. M. (1993). *Relationship between mental health nurses' attitudes toward their patients, caring ability, and sense of power within their work environment.* Unpublished manuscript.

Mayeroff, M. (1971). *On caring.* New York: Harper & Row.

Nkongho, N. (1990). The Caring Ability Inventory. In O. L. Strickland & C. F. Waltz (Eds.), *Measurement of nursing outcomes: Measuring client self-care and coping skills* (Vol. 4), (pp. 3–16). New York: Springer Publishing Co.

Nkongho, N. (1998). *Relationship between ego development and caring ability among college students.* Unpublished manuscript.

Simmons, P. R., & Cavanaugh, S. H. (1996). Relationships among childhood parental care, professional school climate, and nursing student caring ability. *Journal of Professional Nursing, 16,* 373–381.

Simmons, P. R., & Cavanaugh, S. H. (2000). Relationships among student and graduate caring ability and professional school climate. *Journal of Professional Nursing, 16,* 76–83.

APPENDIX: CARING ABILITY INVENTORY

Please read each of the following statements and decide how well it reflects your thoughts and feelings about other people in general. There is no right or wrong answer. Using the response scale, from 1 to 7, circle the degree to which you agree or disagree with each statement directly on the booklet. Please answer all questions.

1	2	3	4	5	6	7
Strongly						Strongly
Disagree						Agree

	Strongly disagree						Strongly agree
	1	2	3	4	5	6	7
1. I believe that learning takes time.	1	2	3	4	5	6	7
2. Today is filled with opportunities.	1	2	3	4	5	6	7
3. I usually say what I mean to others.	1	2	3	4	5	6	7
4. There is very little I can do for a person who is helpless.	1	2	3	4	5	6	7
5. I can see the need for change in myself.	1	2	3	4	5	6	7
6. I am able to like people even if they don't like me.	1	2	3	4	5	6	7
7. I understand people easily.	1	2	3	4	5	6	7
8. I have seen enough in this world for what I need to know.	1	2	3	4	5	6	7
9. I make the time to get to know other people.	1	2	3	4	5	6	7
10. Sometimes I like to be involved, and sometimes I do not like being involved.	1	2	3	4	5	6	7
11. There is nothing I can do to make life better.	1	2	3	4	5	6	7
12. I feel uneasy knowing that another person depends on me.	1	2	3	4	5	6	7
13. I do not like to go out of my way to help other people.	1	2	3	4	5	6	7
14. In dealing with people, it is difficult to let my feelings show.	1	2	3	4	5	6	7
15. It does not matter what I say, as long as I do the correct thing.	1	2	3	4	5	6	7
16. I find it difficult to understand how the other person feels if I have not had similar experiences.	1	2	3	4	5	6	7
17. I admire people who are calm, composed, and patient.	1	2	3	4	5	6	7
18. I believe it is important to accept and respect the attitudes and feelings of others.	1	2	3	4	5	6	7

	Strongly disagree 1 2 3 4 5 6 7	Strongly agree
19. People can count on me to do what I say I will.	1 2 3 4 5 6 7	
20. I believe that there is room for improvement.	1 2 3 4 5 6 7	
21. Good friends look after each other.	1 2 3 4 5 6 7	
22. I find meaning in every situation.	1 2 3 4 5 6 7	
23. I am afraid to let go of those I care for because I am afraid of what might happen to them.	1 2 3 4 5 6 7	
24. I like to offer encouragement to people.	1 2 3 4 5 6 7	
25. I do not like to make commitments beyond the present.	1 2 3 4 5 6 7	
26. I really like myself.	1 2 3 4 5 6 7	
27. I see strengths and weaknesses (limitations) in each individual.	1 2 3 4 5 6 7	
28. New experiences are usually frightening to me.	1 2 3 4 5 6 7	
29. I am afraid to be open and let others see who I am.	1 2 3 4 5 6 7	
30. I accept people just the way they are.	1 2 3 4 5 6 7	
31. When I care for someone else, I do not have to hide my feelings.	1 2 3 4 5 6 7	
32. I do not like to be asked for help.	1 2 3 4 5 6 7	
33. I can express my feelings to people in a warm and caring way.	1 2 3 4 5 6 7	
34. I like talking with people.	1 2 3 4 5 6 7	
35. I regard myself as sincere in my relationships with others.	1 2 3 4 5 6 7	
36. People need space (room, privacy) to think and feel.	1 2 3 4 5 6 7	
37. I can be approached by people at any time.	1 2 3 4 5 6 7	

16

The Postpartum Support Questionnaire

M. Cynthia Logsdon

This chapter presents the Postpartum Support Questionnaire (PSQ), a measure of the amount of social support provided to a woman after childbirth.

PURPOSE

The Postpartum Support Questionnaire (PSQ) is an instrument that measures social support that is provided to a woman after the birth of her baby. Each item of the PSQ is specific to support that a woman commonly needs as she adjusts to parenting and the role of mother. The PSQ can be used any time during the postpartum period, but has most commonly been used at 6 to 8 weeks postpartum. In addition, the PSQ has been used during pregnancy as a measure of predicted postpartum support.

The instrument can be used as an interview guide by researchers, or the woman can complete the instrument on her own. The PSQ was developed for use in clinical settings as a research tool.

CONCEPTUAL BASIS OF THE POSTPARTUM SUPPORT QUESTIONNAIRE

Social support is defined as a well-intentioned action that is given willingly to a person with whom there is a personal relationship and that produces immediate or delayed positive response in the recipient (Hupcey, 1998). Social support has been associated with health and avoidance of disease in research studies since the 1970s (Cassel, 1974). When the measurement of social support has focused on support that is specific to a particular life situation, as opposed to support that the individual receives on a routine basis, the social support scores have been the most predictive of health (Norbeck, 1985). For this reason, the Postpartum Support Questionnaire (PSQ) was developed to specifically measure characteristics of support received during the postpartum period.

The PSQ is based upon the premise that social support has a buffering effect between stress and health or illness outcomes. Social support may slow the release of adrenaline in response to stress (Keeling, Price, Jones, & Harding, 1996). In addition, social support may change the way the stress is viewed, making it less threatening, or increasing feelings of self-esteem or mastery (Thoits, 1986).

In pregnant and postpartum women, social support has been helpful in adapting to the role of mother (Cronenwett, 1985), increasing responsiveness to babies (Crockenberg, 1981), and facilitating the woman's intimate relationship. When the support received matches the support that the woman expected to receive, there is a beneficial effect on the woman's intimate relationship, which in turn results in positive effects on physical and mental well-being (Holmes & Boon, 1990). When support expectations do not match the support received, these "violated expectations" may adversely affect satisfaction with close and intimate relationships (Belsky, 1985), leading to negative influences on the woman's psychosocial status and parenting attitudes (Levitt, 1991). Low social support has been associated with pregnancy complications, labor and delivery complications, infant condition complications (Norbeck & Tilden, 1983), and postpartum depression (Logsdon, McBride, & Birkimer, 1994).

Based on the work of House (1981) and Cronenwett (1985), Logsdon and McBride (1989) classified social support into four categories: material, emotional, informational, and comparison. These four types of support comprise the PSQ and can be defined as follows:

1. Material support is practical assistance including help with meals, laundry, money, and taking over a woman's duties so that she is free for a preferable role.
2. Emotional support consists of encouragement, affection, approval, and feelings of togetherness.
3. Informational support includes sharing information, investigating new sources of information, and helping to solve problems by providing information.
4. Comparison support is that support given by someone in a similar situation, such as another postpartum woman.

PROCEDURES FOR DEVELOPMENT

Items for the PSQ were generated from a review of the literature, from two maternity nursing experts, and from a focus group of postpartum women ($N = 6$). Items generated from both the women and professionals were placed into categories of material, emotional, informational, and comparison support. It was the opinion of the focus group that it was necessary to include in the instrument ratings how important a particular behavior was to the individual, as well as a rating indicating that support had been received. In addition, in order to include the influence of "violated expectations" (e.g., differences in support that a woman expects compared to what she receives), it was decided to survey women in late pregnancy as well as in the postpartum period.

DESCRIPTION

The PSQ consists of 34 items and 4 Likert-type scales. Individual items are assigned to the subscales as follows:

Material support (1, 5, 8, 9, 11, 19, 22, 23, 30)
Emotional support (2, 10, 12, 13, 15, 20, 25, 27, 33, 34)
Informational support (3, 6, 7, 14, 17, 21, 24, 26, 28, 31),
Comparison support (4, 16, 18, 29, 32)

Each of the 34 items asks about importance of support and support expected or received. A response format with 8 options (from *not important* to *very important* and from *no support* to *a lot of support*) is used to measure how important support is expected or (postpartially) perceived to be, and how much help is expected or (postpartially) was received.

ADMINISTRATION AND SCORING

The instrument was designed to be administered either by self-report or by interview. Completion of the instrument takes 10 to 15 minutes. The instrument was developed to be readily comprehensible. Scales are summed separately for importance and support. Total scores can range from 0 to 238 for both importance and support scales. Higher scores indicate higher importance or more support expected (pregnancy) or received (postpartum).

Discrepancy scores were created for both importance and support, and their combination. Discrepancy score 1, change in importance, is the sum of differences between prenatal and postpartum importance ratings of each of the 34 items. This measure balances positive differences against negative ones and reflects any average change in importance for an individual. The second discrepancy score, change in support, is the sum of differences between prenatal and postpartum support ratings on each of the 34 items. This sum reflects any average change in support expected/received. Discrepancy score 3, weighted deviations in support, consists of the absolute value of differences between support expected and received multiplied by prenatal importance (Logsdon et al., 1994). Thus, discrepancy score 3 represents differences in support expected and received combined with the importance rating for all 34 items.

When the PSQ is administered during late pregnancy and at 4 to 6 weeks postpartum, there are five scores that can be correlated with outcome measures (i.e. depression). These scores are importance, support, and three discrepancy scores. When the instrument is given only in the postpartum period, total scores for importance and support are correlated with outcomes.

RELIABILITY AND VALIDITY EVIDENCE

Internal consistency reliability, test-retest reliability, concurrent validity, and construct validity has been demonstrated with the PSQ. In addition to the studies cited in Table 16.1, numerous graduate nursing and psychology students, faculty, and undergraduate students have requested permission to use the PSQ in their research, both nationally and internationally. For example, Wongvisetsirikul (1999) translated the PSQ into the Thai language using nine consultants to determine accuracy and clarity of the translation. Nakajima (2000) has translated the PSQ into Japanese and back into English for use in her doctoral dissertation in nursing. Wittman (2000) has used the PSQ to study the support given by doulas to pregnant and laboring women in British Columbia, Canada.

Internal consistency reliability evidence is also available for the subscales of the PSQ (see Table 16.2). However, in only one study have subscales been used independently of total scores (Davis, Logsdon, & Birkimer, 1996).

CONCLUSIONS AND RECOMMENDATIONS

Researchers have demonstrated strong reliability and validity data for the PSQ in a number of studies. Although the PSQ was developed for use with middle-class, adult women residing in the United States, the instrument has now been used successfully internationally, in women of diverse ages, ethnicity, and socioeconomic status. This point is important for two reasons: Technology makes it possible for scientific results to be shared internationally, resulting in requests by international students and colleagues for instruments to be shared. The PSQ can be recommended in this situation, after appropriate pilot testing. In addition, samples for research studies in the United States must take into account the continuing diversity of the population of this country.

However, the following cautionary note must be given. Social support can be expected to vary by culture in several ways. First, the role expectations for marital partners and other intimate and close relationships

TABLE 16.1 Summary of Psychometrics of Postpartum Support Questionnaire

Study citation	Sample and characteristics	Reliability evidence	Validity evidence
Logsdon & McBride (1989)	Women ($N = 33$) were surveyed prenatally at 36–38 weeks and at 4 weeks postpartum. All women were Caucasian primiparas, married, about 25 years old, and had a mean of 13 years of education.	*Internal consistency:* Alpha scores ranged from .93 to .94 for the total instrument and .51 to .87 for categories of support.	*A priori content validity:* Items were generated using the literature, two maternity nursing experts, and a focus group of postpartum women ($N = 6$).
Logsdon, McBride, & Birkimer (1994)	Women ($N = 105$) were surveyed prenatally at 36 weeks and at 4 weeks postpartum. Women were married, primiparas, Caucasian, about 26 years old, had a mean of 2 years of education past high school, and a semiskilled occupation.	*Internal Consistency:* Alpha scores ranged from .90 to .93 for the total instrument and .72 to .87 by social support categories.	*Factor Analysis:* Exploratory factor analysis with varimax rotation specifying 4 factors resulted in loadings consistent with the original 4 categories of support, with alpha values ranging from .90 to .73 for the categories. Thus, exploratory factor analysis supported the conceptual basis of the measure.
Logsdon & McBride (1991)	Women ($N = 32$) were surveyed at 4 weeks postpartum and at 6 weeks postpartum. Women were	*Internal consistency:* Alpha scores ranged from .88 to .96 for the total instrument and .63 to .94 for	*Concurrent validity:* The PSQ was given concurrently with Part 2 of the PRQ85 (Weinert, 1987).

TABLE 16.1 (*continued*)

Study citation	Sample and characteristics	Reliability evidence	Validity evidence
Logsdon & McBride (1991) (*continued*)	Caucasian, married, 28 years old, and either a semiskilled professional or a housewife.	categories of support. *Test-retest reliability:* Scores ranged from .69 to .79 for total scores and .30 to .79 for categories of support.	Scores were correlated .42 at 4 weeks postpartum and .48 at 6 weeks postpartum, which were mid-range, as expected.
Logsdon, Davis, Birkimer, & Wilkerson (1997)	Women (*N* = 37) were surveyed immediately prior to their premature infant's hospital discharge and at the infant's 4-week neonatal examination. Women were Caucasian, about 26 years old, primiparas, with an average of 13 years of education.	*Internal consistency:* Alpha scores ranged from .92 to .95 for the total instrument and .47 to .93 for categories of support.	
Logsdon, Usui, Birkimer, & McBride (1996)	Data from 4 studies (*N* = 207) were combined for additional analysis.		*Exploratory factor analysis:* Exploratory factor analysis with no number of factors specified resulted in a 7-factor solution. Also estimated were 1-, 4, 5, and 6-factor models, using maximum likelihood (OBLIMIN) rotations. In ex-

TABLE 16.1 *(continued)*

Study citation	Sample and characteristics	Reliability evidence	Validity evidence
Logsdon, Usui, Birkimer, & McBride (1996) *(continued)*			traction with both orthogonal (Varimax) and oblique general, the solutions made sense, but the explained variance was less than 50%. In addition, the determinant of the correlation was quite low (i.e., < .0000000). When examining multicollinearity statistics in the regression procedure, it could have been improved to as "high" as .0000010 by deleting 3 additional items. Because these items seemed conceptually important, they were retained.
			Confirmatory factor analysis: Confirmatory factor analysis using LISREL 7 (Joreskog & Saorbom, 1989) was performed to evaluate the factor structure. Material, emotional, and informational support each divided into 2 parts.

TABLE 16.1 (*continued*)

Study citation	Sample and characteristics	Reliability evidence	Validity evidence
Logsdon, Usui, Birkimer, & McBride (1996) (*continued*)			Item loadings for these subscales are close to what was conceptualized in the original 4-factor model. Although the 4-factor solution best fits the conceptualization of the instrument, when measurement error is correlated, the 2 scales for informational, emotional, and material support are each correlated, yielding an adjusted goodness-of-fit index of .913. Thus, the 7-factor solution can also be conceptualized as a 4-factor model (Logsdon, Usui, Birkimer & McBride, 1996).
Logsdon, Birkimer, & Usui (2000)	Women (*N* = 57) were surveyed at 4–6 weeks postpartum. Women were African American, unmarried, had low incomes, about 20 years old, with an average 11th-grade education.	*Internal consistency:* The alpha scores for the total instrument, both importance and support, were .93.	

TABLE 16.1 (*continued*)

Study citation	Sample and characteristics	Reliability evidence	Validity evidence
Gulick (2000)	Women (*N* = 119) were about 32 years old, with about 15 years of education, and had been diagnosed with multiple sclerosis for 5 years. They were surveyed at 1, 3, and 6 months postpartum, and six months postpartum.	*Internal consistency:* Alpha scores ranged from .89 to .94 for importance and .89 to .94 for support for the total instrument. No alpha scores were cited for categories of support.	None cited.
Wongvisetsirikul (1999)	Women (*N* = 200) were primiparas and resided in Thailand.	*Internal consistency:* The alpha score was .94 for the total instrument (importance and support) and ranged from .75 to .85 for categories of support.	None cited.
Wittman (2000)	Women (*N* = 37) were married, primiparas, of diverse socioeconomic status, approximately 30 years of age, Caucasian, with 12 years of education and residents of Canada. The women were surveyed	*Internal consistency:* Alpha scores for the total instrument were .84 for importance and .89 for support and ranged from .70 to .93 for categories of support.	

TABLE 16.1 (*continued*)

Study citation	Sample and characteristics	Reliability evidence	Validity evidence
Wittman (2000) (*continued*)	4 weeks before delivery and 4 weeks after delivery.		
Nakajima (2000)	Women (*N* = 118) were tested at 1 month postpartum. On average, the women were 32 years old, equally divided between primiparas and multiparas, married, middle class, and well educated.	*Internal consistency:* Alpha scores were .91 for both importance and support for the total instrument. For categories of support, scores ranged from .80 to .91. *Test-retest:* Importance = .54 Support = .81	

TABLE 16.2 Internal Consistency Reliability of Subscales of PSQ

Subscale of Support	Study 1		Study 2		Study 3		Study 4		Study 5	Study 6	Study 7
	Pre-	Post-	Pre-	Post-	Time 1	Time 2	Time 1	Time 2			
Importance of support											
Material											
Emotional	.72	.80	.82	.81	.63	.79	.89	.78	*	.73	.89
Informational	.85	.87	.87	.86	.88	.89	.90	.89	*	.85	.93
Comparison	.72	.64	.80	.79	.81	.87	.82	.86	*	.81	.81
Support expected/received	.83	.70	.72	.88	.78	.89	.68	.65	.85	.87	.87
Material											
Emotional	.54	.77	.81	.80	.77	.89	.80	.87	.75	.79	.86
Informational	.75	.87	.86	.86	.87	.93	.91	.93	.81	.86	.90
Comparison	.51	.76	.83	.80	.77	.86	.76	.88	.76	.82	.88
	.81	.80	.80	.84	.72	.87	.47	.67	.76	.80	.87
	n = 33		*n* = 105		*n* = 32		*n* = 37		*n* = 200	*n* = 118	*n* = 37

Note: Study 1: Logsdon & McBride (1989)

Study 2: Logsdon et al. (1994)

Study 3: Logsdon et al. (1991)

Study 4: Logsdon et al. (1997)

Study 5: Wongvisetsirikul (1999)

Study 6: Nakajima (2000)

Study 7: Wittman (2000)

*Scores are unknown.

vary by culture. This includes how much involvement males have with their partners' pregnancy and parenting, including the amount and type of support provided to their partners. Second, role expectations for new mothers vary by culture, including how independently the mother is expected to function at various intervals of time. Third, there is variation by culture of the importance of the individual compared to the group. Women may not feel free to express their needs for support in a culture where the importance of the group is paramount (Logsdon, 2000).

The PSQ is an instrument developed to measure social support. Social support should be differentiated from support provided by professionals or paraprofessionals. As Wittman (2000) determined in her study of pregnant women and doulas, additional items may be necessary if the instrument is used outside of its intended purpose.

The boundaries of the usefulness of the PSQ should continue to be tested. Longitudinal studies should determine the length of time that the PSQ items are relevant as descriptors of support that is important, expected and received. Statistical analysis should include scores on the PSQ that are predictive of particular outcomes. Additional outcomes, which are the result of inadequate social support, should be studied. There is a need to explore subscales of the PSQ as predictors of outcomes, particularly how these subscales vary within cultures.

In summary, for the past 10 years the PSQ has been a useful instrument to measure social support in postpartum women. The science in this area can be advanced by following the recommendations above.

REFERENCES

Belsky, J. (1985). Exploring individual differences in marital change across the transition to parenthood: The role of violated expectations. *Journal of Marriage and the Family, 47*, 1037–1044.

Cassel, J. (1974). The contribution of the social environment to host resistance: The fourth Wade Hampton Frost lecture. *American Journal of Epidemiology, 104*, 107–123.

Crockenberg, S. B. (1981). Infant irritability, mother responsiveness, and social influences on the security of infant-mother attachment. *Child Development, 52*, 857–865.

Cronenwett, L. R. (1985). Network structure, social support, and psychological outcomes of pregnancy. *Nursing Research, 34*, 93–99.

Davis, D. W., Logsdon, M. C., & Birkimer, J. C. (1996). Types of support expected and received by mothers after their infant's discharge from the NICU. *Issues in Comprehensive Pediatric Nursing, 19*, 263–273.

Gulick, E. (2000). The effects of infant feeding method and postpartum support on the health of mothers with multiple sclerosis.

Holmes, J. G., & Boon, S. D. (1990). Developments in the field of close relationships: Creating foundations for intervention strategies. *Personality and Social Psychology Bulletin, 16,* 23–41.

House, J. S. (1981). *Work stress and social support.* Reading, MA: Addison-Wesley.

Hupcey, J. E. (1998). Social support: Assessing conceptual coherence. *Qualitative Health Research, 8,* 304–318.

Joreskog, K. G., & Saorbom, D. (1989). *LISREL: Analysis of linear structural relationships by the method of maximum likelihood* (Version 7). Mooresville, IN: Scientific Software.

Keeling, D. I., Price, P. E., Jones, E., & Harding, K. G. (1996). Social support: Some pragmatic implications for health care professionals. *Journal of Advanced Nursing, 23,* 76–81.

Levitt, M. J. (1991). Attachment and close relationships: A life span perspective. In J. L. Gewirtz & W. M. Kurtines (Eds.), *Intersections with attachment* (pp. 183–206). Hillsdale, NJ: Earlbaum.

Logsdon, M. C. (2000). *Social support for pregnant and postpartum women.* AWHONN monograph.

Logsdon, M. C., Birkimer, J. C., & Usui, W. M. (2000). The link of social support and postpartum depression in African-American women with low incomes. *Maternal–Child Nursing, 25,* 262–266.

Logsdon, M. C., Davis, D. W., Birkimer, J. C., & Wilkerson, S. A. (1997). Predictors of depression in mothers of preterm infants. *Journal of Social Behavior and Personality, 12,* 73–88.

Logsdon, M. C., & McBride, A. B. (1989). Help after childbirth: Do women get what they expect and need? *Kentucky Nurse, 37,* 14–15.

Logsdon, M. C., & McBride, A. B. (1991). Further data on the postpartum support questionnaire. *Kentucky Nurse, 39,* 13.

Logsdon, M. C., McBride, A. B., & Birkimer, J. C. (1994). Social support and postpartum depression. *Research in Nursing and Health, 17,* 449–457.

Logsdon, M. C., & Usui, W. M. (2001). Psychosocial predictors of postpartum depression in diverse groups of women. *Western Journal of Nursing Research, 23*(6), 563–574.

Logsdon, M. C., Usui, W. M., Birkimer, J. C., & McBride, A. B. (1996). The postpartum support questionnaire: Reliability and validity. *Journal of Nursing Measurement, 4,* 129–142.

Nakajima, T. (2000). *Social support in Japanese postpartum women.* Unpublished manuscript.

Norbeck, J. S. (1985). Types and sources of social support for managing job stress in critical care nursing. *Nursing Research, 34,* 225–230.

Norbeck, J. S., & Tilden, V. P. (1983). Life stress, social support, and emotional disequilibrium in complications of pregnancy: A prospective multivariate study. *Journal of Health and Social Behavior, 24,* 30–46.

Thoits, P. A. (1986). Conceptual, methodological, and theoretical problems in studying social support as a buffer against life stress. *Journal of Health and Social Behavior, 23,* 145–159.

Weinert, C. (1987). A social support measure: PRQ85. *Nursing Research, 36,* 273–277.

Wittman, L. (2000). *Doulas, social support, and postpartum depression.* Unpublished master's thesis. Trinity Western University, British Columbia, Canada.

Wongvisetsirikul, P. (1999). *Postpartum support in Thai women.* Unpublished manuscript.

APPENDIX: POSTPARTUM SUPPORT QUESTIONNAIRE

TODAY'S DATE:

The following questions ask about ways in which you have needed help since your baby was born. First, each question asks you to indicate how *IMPORTANT* this type of help was for you. Then, you are to indicate *HOW MUCH* help you received with this item. Please circle the number of the response that best describes your feeling or opinion.

	IMPORTANT NEED		HELP RECEIVED	
	Not important 0	Very Important 7	No help 0	Lot of help 7
1. Needed help with cooking meals.	0 1 2 3 4 5 6 7		0 1 2 3 4 5 6 7	
2. Needed to be reassured that I was more than just someone's mother.	0 1 2 3 4 5 6 7		0 1 2 3 4 5 6 7	
3. Needed to have information on taking care of my own body as it heals following the birth of my baby.	0 1 2 3 4 5 6 7		0 1 2 3 4 5 6 7	
4. Needed to talk to another new mother about my baby's behavior.	0 1 2 3 4 5 6 7		0 1 2 3 4 5 6 7	
5. Needed help with laundry.	0 1 2 3 4 5 6 7		0 1 2 3 4 5 6 7	
6. Needed to have information on which skin rashes were normal for the baby to have.	0 1 2 3 4 5 6 7		0 1 2 3 4 5 6 7	
7. Needed to know if my baby's sleeping patterns were normal.	0 1 2 3 4 5 6 7		0 1 2 3 4 5 6 7	
8. Needed help in taking care of my baby so that I could take a shower, eat, or have some time to myself.	0 1 2 3 4 5 6 7		0 1 2 3 4 5 6 7	
9. Needed to have time for friends and activities (exercise, sports, clubs, parties) I used to enjoy.	0 1 2 3 4 5 6 7		0 1 2 3 4 5 6 7	
10. Needed for others to act as if I am special.	0 1 2 3 4 5 6 7		0 1 2 3 4 5 6 7	
11. Needed help in cleaning the house/apartment.	0 1 2 3 4 5 6 7		0 1 2 3 4 5 6 7	
12. Needed for others to appreciate my care of the baby.	0 1 2 3 4 5 6 7		0 1 2 3 4 5 6 7	

	IMPORTANT NEED		HELP RECEIVED	
	Not important 0	Very Important 7	No help 0	Lot of help 7
13. Needed to have others act as if my ideas, decisions, and ways of doing things were right or acceptable.	0 1 2 3 4 5 6 7		0 1 2 3 4 5 6 7	
14. Needed to have information on what my my baby's bowel movements should look like.	0 1 2 3 4 5 6 7		0 1 2 3 4 5 6 7	
15. Needed for others to act like it is okay for me to need help.	0 1 2 3 4 5 6 7		0 1 2 3 4 5 6 7	
16. Needed to talk with another new mother about how to do baby care.	0 1 2 3 4 5 6 7		0 1 2 3 4 5 6 7	
17. Needed to have information on resuming sex and/ or birth control.	0 1 2 3 4 5 6 7		0 1 2 3 4 5 6 7	
18. Needed to talk with another new mother about how I was adjusting to the role of mother.	0 1 2 3 4 5 6 7		0 1 2 3 4 5 6 7	
19. Needed help in obtaining more sleep for me.	0 1 2 3 4 5 6 7		0 1 2 3 4 5 6 7	
20. Needed for someone to talk with me and listen to me about what is interesting and important to me.	0 1 2 3 4 5 6 7		0 1 2 3 4 5 6 7	
21. Needed to have information on breastfeeding.	0 1 2 3 4 5 6 7		0 1 2 3 4 5 6 7	
22. Needed help in going to the grocery or drugstore.	0 1 2 3 4 5 6 7		0 1 2 3 4 5 6 7	
23. Needed for someone to watch my baby so that I could have time alone together with my partner/ boyfriend.	0 1 2 3 4 5 6 7		0 1 2 3 4 5 6 7	
24. Needed to have information on my baby's crying (why the baby cries and how to comfort him/her).	0 1 2 3 4 5 6 7		0 1 2 3 4 5 6 7	
25. Needed for others to take my worries and concerns seriously.	0 1 2 3 4 5 6 7		0 1 2 3 4 5 6 7	

	IMPORTANT NEED			HELP RECEIVED		
	Not important 0		Very Important 7	No help 0		Lot of help 7
26. Needed to have information on handling stress and/ or discomfort.	0 1 2 3 4 5 6 7			0 1 2 3 4 5 6 7		
27. Needed for others to reassure me that I was not alone in being responsible for my baby.	0 1 2 3 4 5 6 7			0 1 2 3 4 5 6		
28. Needed to have information on how to care for my baby's umbilical cord (navel, belly button).	0 1 2 3 4 5 6 7			0 1 2 3 4 5 6 7		
29. Needed to talk with another new mother about the best places to get baby care supplies, clothing, etc., needed.	0 1 2 3 4 5 6 7			0 1 2 3 4 5 6 7		
30. Needed money for baby equipment, supplies, supplies, or bills that go along with having my baby.	0 1 2 3 4 5 6 7			0 1 2 3 4 5 6 7		
31. Needed to have information on my baby's hiccups (why the baby hiccups and what to do).	0 1 2 3 4 5 6 7			0 1 2 3 4 5 6 7		
32. Needed to talk with another new mother about my labor and delivery experience.	0 1 2 3 4 5 6 7			0 1 2 3 4 5 6 7		
33. Needed for others to touch, kiss, and hug me.	0 1 2 3 4 5 6 7			0 1 2 3 4 5 6 7		
34. Needed to have others treat me like I am responsible and competent.	0 1 2 3 4 5 6 7			0 1 2 3 4 5 6 7		

Note: Dr. M. Cynthia Logsdon holds the copyright for the PSQ. Please contact her for permission to use.

17

The Long-Term Quality of Life Instrument for Female Cancer Survivors

Gwen Wyatt and Laurie Friedman Donze

This chapter discusses the Long-Term Quality of Life Instrument, a measure of quality of life in long-term female cancer survivors.

PURPOSE

The Long-Term Quality of Life (LTQL) instrument was developed to enhance the new generation of quality of life instruments by specifically assessing quality of life of the long-term female cancer survivor in multiple domains of life, including the often omitted domain of spirituality (Gotay & Muraoka, 1998). The LTQL measures four constructs within the concept of quality of life: somatic concerns, spiritual/philosophical views of life, fitness, and social support. The instrument was designed for use among female survivors of various cancers, with a length of survivorship of at least 5 years. The LTQL was initially tested on participants obtained from a hospital tumor registry. It was designed to be administered by mail and completed at home; however, the LTQL is appropriate for use in a clinical setting, such as a hospital or clinic, with women who may or may not be receiving current medical care or other supportive services.

CONCEPTUAL FRAMEWORK

Quality of life is often conceptualized as a multidimensional construct, but there is not consensus in the literature on the specific dimensions of quality of life (Padilla, Grant, & Ferrell, 1992). Quality of life is broadly defined by a wide range of physical and psychological characteristics and limitations that describe an individual's ability to function and derive satisfaction from life (Walker, 1987). Health-related quality of life "generally applies to the level of well-being and satisfaction associated with an individual's life and how this is affected by disease, accidents, and treatments" (Grant, Padilla, Ferrell, & Rhiner, 1990, p. 260). Current practice shows a tendency to qualify the term by speaking of health-related quality of life when referring to individuals responding to the effects of disease and treatment (Padilla et al., 1992). In this chapter, the terms *quality of life* and *health-related quality of life* are used interchangeably, referring to a multidimensional interaction of life domains (bio-psycho-social-spiritual), with emphasis on physical concerns, social support needs, health behaviors and beliefs, and spiritual/philosophical issues (Wyatt & Friedman, 1996).

The Ferrell (1993) quality of life model for women with breast cancer, on which the current instrument was based, consists of four domains: physical well-being, encompassing areas such as symptom management; psychological well-being, covering concerns such as fear of recurrence, anxiety, and depression; the social concerns domain, including altered family and friendship roles and relationships; and spiritual well-being, addressing the meaning of illness, religious beliefs, and heightened awareness of mortality as a result of cancer. The four major concepts measured by the LTQL were based on these domains of quality of life.

Ferrell and colleagues (Ferrell, Dow, & Grant, 1995; Ferrell, Dow, Leigh, Ly, & Gulasekaram, 1995) expanded the 1993 model by revising their quality of life instrument to be tested with other cancer survivors. The length of survivorship among their sample ranged from 4 months to 28 years, with a mean survival of 5.7 years. Testing of the revised version of their instrument (the QOL-CS) supported the importance of including the spiritual domain along with the physical, social, and psychological domains.

In developing a quality of life instrument, we chose to follow the course set by Grant and associates (1992), Ferrell (1993), and Dow and colleagues (Dow, Ferrell, Leigh, Ly, & Gulasekaram, 1996), who included existential as well as religious beliefs and attitudes in the spiritual domain, while attempting to keep the life domains broad. Using the four domains from the Ferrell (1993) framework, instrument development and subsequent item generation began with focus group discussions in which the goal was to be completely open to the survivors' areas of interest and concern. Thus, the LTQL built on previous work on quality of life measures, while enhancing those measures by allowing long-term female cancer survivors to shape and define the dimensions most relevant to their lives. Furthermore, we sought to refine and strengthen the spirituality/existential domain, which, to date, has received less attention than other quality of life dimensions. Finally, unlike the studies by Ferrell and colleagues (Ferrell et al., 1995; Ferrell, Dow, Leigh, etc al., 1995), we focused on long-term survivors of 5 years or longer. The LTQL measures four concepts based on Ferrell's quality of life domains. Somatic concerns relate to physical considerations resulting from the woman's cancer experience with a social-emotional component. A spiritual/philosophical view of life is an attitude that reflects an increased insight and appreciation for life since the illness. The concept, fitness, relates to the woman's behavior and beliefs about exercise. Finally, social support reflects the woman's need for support and desire to be of service to others.

PROCEDURES FOR DEVELOPMENT

The process of developing the LTQL instrument was "qualitative to quantitative," in which the analysis of focus group transcripts was used to assess the expressed concerns and issues of long-term female survivors. Broad, open-ended questions were asked based on Ferrell's (1993) domains of quality of life (see Wyatt, Kurtz, & Liken, 1993, for a complete review of the focus group process and outcomes), and 13 content areas were generated. A minimum of five items for each of the content areas was then written, with each statement reflecting an attribute of the content area.

Content validity was assessed by submitting all items to an independent senior research team consisting of three researchers. The judges were asked to determine whether the items fit appropriately into the categories for which they were written, whether any other items should be included in each category, and whether the range of possible items was covered. The team of judges also gave feedback on wording, readability, and the appropriateness and comprehensiveness of statements for each content domain. In addition, one focus group participant, who was also a nurse, was asked to provide feedback about wording and content of the items.

Following administration of the instrument, exploratory factor analyses were conducted to compare statistically generated factors to the original dimensions developed from the focus groups. An unrestricted principal components factor analysis (Dunteman, 1989) with a varimax rotation was run on the 67 items, and a criterion of less than .60 was used to eliminate items of lower (than "mediocre") sampling adequacy (Kaiser, 1974), resulting in an improved set of 39 items with a mean sampling adequacy of .85.

A second unrestricted principal components analysis with a varimax rotation was performed on the 39 remaining items, resulting in nine factors with eigenvalues greater than 1. Based on an examination of the factor scree plot and the percent of variance accounted for by each factor, the analysis was repeated with a restriction to four factors, to account for more than 50% of the variance. Five items were deleted from this new 4-factor solution due to low (< .40) factor loadings or loading comparably on more than one factor. These 4 factors, accounting for 53% of the total variance, comprise the LTQL's subscales.

DESCRIPTION

The LTQL consists of 34 items assessing multiple content areas from the focus group discussions, including body image, apparel, pain, exercise, change in senses, change in social support, desire to be of service to others, susceptibility to cancer, change in perception of health and illness, spiritual guidance for health decisions, and change in philosophical view of life. Approximately 60% of the items are worded positively to reflect increased quality of life, with 40% worded negatively to reflect decreased quality of life. The 34 items are rated on a 5-point scale, to assess the extent to which the item applies to the respondent: 0 (*not at all*), 1 (*a little*), 2 (*a fair amount*), 3 (*much*), and 4 (*very much*). The LTQL items are organized into 4 subscales, based on the factor analysis: Somatic Concerns (14 items), Spiritual/Philosophical Views of Life (11 items), Fitness (5 items), and Social Support (4 items).

ADMINISTRATION AND SCORING

The LTQL was designed to be administered by mail. It is a questionnaire that can be completed by respondents in their own homes with little explanation. The LTQL is scored by totaling the numeric scores on each of the four subscales and dividing by the number of items in each scale, resulting in mean subscale scores. The potential range of mean subscale scores is 0 to 4, although actual mean scores are likely to fall somewhere within this range. High scores on items or subscales (i.e., 4) indicate that the item or subscale, reflecting a concern or change since the cancer, applies to the respondent "very much." Conversely, a subscale mean of 0 signifies that the subscale applies "not at all." Because items are worded both positively and negatively, on some items, a high score (i.e., 4) would be indicative of high quality of life, whereas on others, a score of 4 would indicate low quality of life. However, all items are coded to reflect a negative result of the cancer experience, or impaired quality of life post-cancer. Therefore, scores on the 21 positively worded items (reflecting positive changes or effects) are reversed to reflect negative quality of life to be consistent with scoring of other similar instruments. Table 17.1 presents the items and indicates those that are reverse-scored.

RELIABILITY AND VALIDITY

Subscale Reliabilities

In the original testing of the LTQL with 188 long-term female cancer survivors, internal consistency estimates were calculated for each of the

TABLE 17.1 Long-Term Quality of Life (LTQL) Items and Reverse Scoring

Item number	Reverse-scored	Long-Term Quality of Life items
1	*	I think I could be helpful to others who have recently been diagnosed with cancer.
2	*	I have a better idea about what serious illness is since having had cancer.
3	*	I feel a guiding energy in my life which has my best interest in mind.
4	*	Exercise helps me feel healthy.
5	*	I am satisfied with my body as it is now.
6	*	I would like to be a resource person to others who have recently been diagnosed with cancer.
7		I feel more susceptible to other illnesses since having had cancer.
8		I am self-conscious about my body since my cancer.
9	*	Since having had cancer, I have a greater appreciation for the time I spend with my friends and family.
10	*	I follow my inner voice when making health decisions .
11		I have to raise my arm or foot on a pillow so my rings or shoes fit all day since my cancer treatment .
12		I have difficulty finding suitable clothing since my cancer.
13	*	I have intuitive experiences that reassure me about my health care choices.
14		I continue to have pain since my cancer treatment.
15	*	I exercise more frequently.
16	*	I receive subtle cues that give me confidence in my health decisions.
17	*	Regular exercise keeps me healthy, so I am less likely to get cancer again.
18	*	I am sympathetic with family/friends who have major illnesses, such as heart or kidney disease since my cancer.
19		I feel dissatisfied with the way I look since my cancer.
20	*	Since having had cancer, I tend to notice things in nature more, such as sunsets, raindrops, and spring flowers.

TABLE 17.1 *(continued)*

Item number	Reverse-scored	Long-Term Quality of Life items
21	*	Exercise helps decrease my fatigue.
22		My eyesight has gotten worse since my cancer treatment.
23		I have difficulty finding suitable clothing since my cancer.
24		My social life is less satisfying since having cancer.
25		In the past week, I have experienced pain related to having had cancer.
26	*	I feel an inner direction that helps me make wise decisions.
27	*	I have become closer with some family members/friends since having had cancer.
28		I have had numbness and/or tingling since my cancer treatment.
29	*	Exercise helps me feel energetic.
30	*	Since having had cancer, I don't take life's little things for granted
31	*	I would find it beneficial to speak with other long-term cancer survivors.
32		I frequently feel distressed with pain/discomfort because it reminds me of my cancer.
33	*	I think that I have support and understanding to offer other long-term survivors.
34		I have had to adjust the way I exercise since my cancer.

four subscales using Cronbach's alpha. Subscale composite scores were computed as the average of individual item scores on that subscale. Reliabilities of the four subscales ranged from .87 to .92. To correct for multiple correlations, a minimum *p*-value of .008 was used to determine significance (.05 ÷ 6 = .008). The significant interscale correlations suggest that the subscales all measure components of an underlying quality of life construct. Test–retest reliability was not assessed because of the lack of repeated questionnaire administration.

Content Validity

Content validity of the LTQL items was initially assessed by interrater agreement on subscale items derived from focus group coding categories.

Content validity was further supported by conceptual congruence between the four subscales of the LTQL and Ferrell's (1993) original four quality of life domains.

Concurrent Validity

Concurrent validity was assessed by comparing the LTQL with the Cancer Rehabilitation Evaluation System–Short Form (CaRES-SF), an established measure of quality of life (Schag, Ganz, & Heinrich, 1991). A minimum p-value of .002 was used to determine significance, to correct for multiple correlations (.05 ÷ 30 = .002). The somatic concerns factor was significantly correlated with all of the CaRES subscales (Physical, Medical, Psychosocial, Sexual, and Marital). Fitness was significantly correlated with the CaRES Physical subscale. Finally, the total LTQL score was highly correlated with all CaRES subscales (except Marital), and with the CaRES total score.

Construct Validity

Construct validity was assessed by one-way analyses of variance, comparing differences between subscale means according to demographic and health status variables. Subscale composite scores differed as expected based on the women's characteristics.

As would be expected, among breast cancer survivors, mastectomy patients reported a lower quality of life on the somatic subscale and the total scale than did lumpectomy patients ($t = 3.73$, $p < .001$; $t = 2.38$, p .05, respectively). Also, women currently experiencing a recurrence of any cancer reported higher somatic concerns and lower overall quality of life than those not currently experiencing a recurrence ($t = 4.65$, $p < .001$; $t = 1.95$, $p < .05$, respectively). Furthermore, those with the longest survival time (11 or more years) reported lower quality of life with regard to somatic concerns than did women of shorter survival time ($t = 2.74$, $p < .05$). Although this result may appear counterintuitive, it should be noted that length of survival was significantly related to recurrence status, with the longer-term survivors more likely to have experienced a recurrence, either currently or previously.

Lumpectomy patients reported significantly higher scores on the fitness subscale than did breast cancer survivors who received mastectomies ($t = 2.78$, $p < .05$). In the whole sample, the youngest women (age 22 to 39) reported lower quality of life than did the older women ($t = 2.18$, $p < .05$) on spiritual/philosophical views of life. On the social support subscale, women who had never experienced a recurrence reported significantly lower support than those experiencing a current recurrence ($t = $

2.18, $p < .05$). As such, the longer-term survivors (being more likely to have experienced a recurrence) reported significantly higher levels of social support than shorter-term survivors ($t = 2.10$, $p < .05$).

Recent Testing

Since the original testing of the LTQL, the Spiritual/Philosophical subscale has been used most often without the other subscales most often. This subscale represents a construct that is not readily available in other quality of life measures. In 1999, Wyatt, Friedman, Given, Given, and Beckrow reported on the Spiritual/Philosophical subscale in a population of older cancer patients. The sample for this study of 699 participants (the majority were men) had a mean age of 72 years. Most had stage 1 or 2 cancers and were in active treatment. The Spiritual/Philosophical subscale alpha reliability for this sample was .78.

Another study-in-progress is using the Spirituality/Philosophical subscale (Given, Wyatt, & Given, 2000). This study's sample consists of cancer patients in active treatment. The study is open to both men and women, but the majority are women with breast cancer. Based on Wave I data, the alpha coefficient is .77 ($n = 71$); incomplete Wave II data currently have an alpha of .86 ($n = 51$). This study will eventually provide information on test-retest reliability for this subscale.

Both of these studies demonstrate adequate reliability when used with male and female patients during active treatment. Further testing may show that this LTQL subscale is more universal than its original intent (i.e., a measure for 5 year and longer female survivors).

A third study will be testing all four subscales of the LTQL with breast cancer survivors who are 20 to 30 weeks postdiagnosis (Wyatt & Collins, 2000). This research will shed more light on the instrument's usefulness during the post-active-treatment period. Reliabilities are yet to be assessed for this sample.

In addition to the studies cited above, 15 investigators have requested a copy of the full LTQL instrument and scoring instructions, but have either not yet used it or have not yet analyzed the data. Therefore, additional information on the LTQL's reliability and validity should be forthcoming.

CONCLUSIONS AND RECOMMENDATIONS

The results of this research support the potential of the LTQL to be a useful measure of quality of life in long-term female cancer survivors. An exploratory principal components factor analysis of the LTQL produced 4 distinct factors with factor loadings of greater than .40 and subscale reliabilities ranging from 0.87 to 0.92. These factors are congruent with Ferrell's theoretical domains of quality of life developed for women with breast cancer. Although the LTQL retained all four of Ferrell's domains of quality of life (physical, psychological, social, and spiritual) within one instrument, individual items were reconfigured to demonstrate a complexity of overlapping domains helpful in understanding quality of life in the long-term female cancer survivor.

The strength of the LTQL is that it is a multidimensional assessment tool applicable to the long-term cancer survivor. Unlike some other quality of life instruments, the LTQL evaluates quality of life as related to spirituality, in addition to the biopsychosocial domains. The LTQL is short, easy to administer, and easy to score. The instrument may, however, be limited in the content domains that it assesses. Future research may seek to include and test additional subscales to make the LTQL more comprehensive.

Further research to refine the current version of the LTQL should include the assessment of additional external variables on which women would be expected to differ, to further support construct validity. Factor stability should be assessed by performing a confirmatory factor analysis using an independent sample of participants. Test–retest reliability and discriminant validity should be confirmed. Testing of the LTQL with a sample more representative of minorities is also needed. In addition, the utility of the instrument with samples of less than 5 years' survival time, those in active treatment, and men needs further exploration, and may ultimately add insight on the breadth of the potential application of the LTQL.

Scores on each of the four subscales indicate areas of possible diminished quality of life, which can be used to guide treatment recommendations for cancer patients who may or may not be currently receiving cancer care or other supportive services. More broadly, data collected from the LTQL could be used to inform program development for long-term cancer survivors. When further testing of this instrument is completed, the LTQL may prove useful in studying long-term cancer survivors longitudinally, to assess changes in quality of life over time. The overlapping of life domains in the LTQL subscales may provide clues as to how best to intervene with the long-term survivor. The LTQL could also be used as a pre-intervention or needs-assessment instrument, and finally, as a post-intervention evaluation tool for programs targeting long-term cancer survivors.

AUTHORS' NOTE

The data presented in this chapter were also reported on in the following related publications: "Breast Cancer Survivors: An Exploration of Quality of Life Issues" by Wyatt et al. (1993); "Psychological and Sexual Well-Being, Philosophical/Spiritual Views, and Health Habits of Long-Term Cancer Survivors" by Kurtz and Wyatt (1995); "Preliminary Testing of the Long-Term Quality of Life (LTQL) Instrument for Female Cancer Survivors" by Wyatt et al. (1996); "Development and Testing of a Quality of Life Model for Long-Term Female Cancer Survivors" by Wyatt and Friedman (1996); and "Long-Term Female Cancer Survivors: Quality of Life Issues and Clinical Implications" by Wyatt and Friedman (1996). This research was supported by Bristol-Myers through the Oncology Nursing Society, Gwen Wyatt, Principal Investigator. We wish to thank Barbara Given, RN, PhD, FAAN, Charles Given, PhD, and Manfred Stommel, PhD for serving as our panel of experts during instrument development.

REFERENCES

Dow, K. H., Ferrell, B. R., Leigh, S., Ly, J., & Gulasekaram, P. (1996). An evaluation of the quality of life among long-term survivors of breast cancer. *Breast Cancer Research and Treatment, 39,* 261–273.

Dunteman, G. H. (1989). *Principal components analysis.* Beverly Hills, CA: Sage.

Ferrell, B. R. (1993). Overview of breast cancer: Quality of life. *Oncology Patient Care, 3*(3), 7–8.

Ferrell, B.R., Dow, K.H., & Grant, M. (1995a). Measurement of the quality of life in cancer survivors. *Quality of Life Research, 4,* 523–31.

Ferrell, B. R., Dow, K. H., Leigh, S., Ly, J., & Gulasekaram, P. (1995b). Quality of life in long-term cancer survivors. *Oncology Nursing Forum, 22,* 915–922.

Given, C., Wyatt, G., & Given, B. (2000). *Complementary therapy use among cancer patients while receiving chemotherapy.* Unpublished manuscript.

Gotay, C., & Muraoka, M. (1998). Quality of life in long-term survivors of adult-onset cancers. *Journal of the National Cancer Institute, 90,* 656–667.

Grant, M., Ferrell, B., Schmidt, G.M., Fonbuena, P., Niland, J. C., & Forman, S. J. (1992). Measurement of quality of life in bone marrow transplantation survivors. *Quality of Life Research, 1,* 375–388.

Grant, M. M., Padilla, G. V., Ferrell, B. R., & Rhiner, M. (1990). Assessment of quality of life with a single instrument. *Seminars in Oncology Nursing, 6,* 260–270.

Kaiser, H. F. (1974). An index of factorial simplicity. *Psychometrika, 39,* 31–36.

Padilla, G. V., Grant, M. M., & Ferrell, B. (1992). Nursing research into quality of life. *Quality of Life Research, 1,* 341–348.

Schag, C. A. C., Ganz, P. A., & Heinrich, R. (1991). Cancer Rehabilitation Evaluation System-Short Form (CARES-SF). *Cancer, 68,* 1406–1413.

Walker, C. S. (1987). *Quality of life: Assessment and applications.* London: MTP Press.

Wyatt, G., & Collins, C. (2000). *A rehabilitation program for women following breast cancer surgery.* Unpublished manuscript.

Wyatt, G., Friedman, L., Given, C., Given, B., & Beckrow, K. (1999). Complementary therapy use among older cancer patients. *Cancer Practice, 7,* 136–144.

Wyatt, G., Kurtz, M. E., Friedman, L.L., Given, G., Given, C. W. (1996) Preliminary testing of the Long-Term Quality of Life (LTQL) instrument for female cancer survivors. Journal of Nursing Measurement, 4(2), 153–170.

Wyatt, G. K. H., & Friedman, L. (1996). Long-term female cancer survivors: Quality of life issues and clinical implications. *Cancer Nursing, 19,* 1–7.

Wyatt, G. K. H., Kurtz, M. E., & Liken, M. (1993). Breast cancer survivors: An exploration of quality of life issues. *Cancer Nursing, 6,* 440–448.

PART IV
Measuring Health Behaviors

18

The Multidimensional Health Behavior Inventory

Pamela A. Kulbok, Kimberly F. Carter, Joan H. Baldwin, Mattia J. Gilmartin, and Bessie Kirkwood

This chapter discusses the Multidimensional Health Behavior Inventory, a measure of health behaviors for older adolescents and young adults.

PURPOSE

Health promotion strategies to instigate healthy and reduce risky behaviors in young people often yield minimal success because of complex behavior patterns and limited knowledge of the structure of health behaviors (Donovan, Jessor, & Costa, 1993; Elliott, 1993; Kulbok, Earls, & Montgomery, 1988). The Multidimensional Health Behavior Inventory (MHBI) was developed to measure health behaviors for older adolescents and young adults. The psychometric properties of the MHBI and the structure of a wide variety of health promotion behaviors were successfully evaluated with data from a college population of older adolescents and young adults (Kulbok, Carter, Baldwin, Gilmartin, & Kirkwood, 1999). This psychometric work built on previous research with high school and college students and expanded the number and type of behaviors studied. The intent was to identify the structure of a broad range of health behaviors that emerge in college, which may or may not be different from those behaviors of young and middle adolescence and noncollege students.

CONCEPTUAL FRAMEWORK

The framework, which guided development of the MHBI, is the resource model of health behavior (Kulbok, 1985a). The conceptual basis for the model was developed through critical review of health behavior literature and research (Kulbok, 1983; Kulbok & Baldwin, 1992; Kulbok, Baldwin, Cox, & Duffy, 1997). The resource model proposes that health is a positive, multidimensional process, that health status and perceptions of health influence behavior, and that definition and measurement of health behavior is directed by the researcher's implicit or explicit definition of health. The major concepts within the resource model are social resources, health resources, and health behavior.

In an early test of the resource model using adult data from a national survey, Kulbok (1985a) examined the association among social resources, health resources, and health behaviors. Education and income were social resources; the components of health resources and health behaviors were identified using principal components factor analysis. The three health resource factors were activity level, general well-being, and health comparison. The five health behavior factors were dental, checkup, harmful consumption, health protection, and fitness. Two resource model variables, higher education and health comparison, predicted all five health behavior factors. However, the major study findings supported the propositions that health behaviors do have multiple dimensions and that different types of health behaviors may have different correlates or causes. A series of studies have followed this initial work to further identify clustering patterns and interrelationships of the health behaviors in different populations (Kulbok, 1985b; Kulbok, Cary, & Seifert, 1991; Kulbok et al., 1988; Kulbok, Earls, Robins, & Jung, 1985; Kulbok, Earls, Robins, Stiffman, & Jung, 1985; Kurtenbach, 1992). Building on this conceptual and empirical base, the investigators have developed a new tool to measure a wide variety of health promotion behaviors in young people. The ultimate goal of this research is to use the MHBI to develop and test innovative, age-appropriate, and behavior-specific health promotion strategies.

PROCEDURES FOR DEVELOPMENT OF THE MHBI

The MHBI is a norm-referenced or discriminative index that measures self-reported health and risk behaviors. Concept analysis (Kulbok, 1983; Kulbok & Baldwin, 1992), empirical research (Kulbok, 1985a; Kulbok et al., 1988), and a content validity study (Kulbok et al., 1997) provided the foundation for instrument development. Health promotion behavior is any action undertaken by an individual that improves or promotes health and well-being and includes both positive health-oriented actions and negative avoidance behaviors (Kulbok et al., 1997). This definition guided the selection of 105 behavioral items from the literature and existing health behavior scales in the public domain. The MHBI was designed to have distinct dimensions or scales, rather than a total summative scale. Health behavior categories were identified, including nutrition, substance use/avoidance, exercise/fitness, personal health–emotional/social, personal health–physical, dental behavior, environmental health and safety, and general health care. Theoretical and empirical support for these dimensions is inconsistent; therefore, the specific number and type of dimensions for the MHBI were derived using factor analytic procedures.

Five health promotion research experts evaluated the content validity of the 105 item stems by judging whether each item in the MHBI was behavioral and the "relevance to health" of each item. The content validity scale was a 4-point rating scale, that measured the relevance to health of the behavioral items, ranging from 1 (*irrelevant*) to 4 (*extremely relevant*). Items reported to be "irrelevant" by 50% or more of the experts were deleted and items reported to be "extremely relevant" by 50% or more of the experts were accepted for the tool. Items that did not meet this criterion had to have a mean of greater than or equal to 2.5 to be retained for the instrument (Campbell-Grossman, Pozehl, & Zimmerman, 1996; Zimmerman & Westfall, 1985).

Thirty young adults ranging in age from 15 to 24 years assessed questionnaire administration favorably. The overall tool was reevaluated for adequacy of domain sampling by the investigators and an outside consultant. Items measuring diet, substance use/avoidance, and sexual activity were underrepresented in the original inventory. The MHBI was expanded to 125 items to ensure inclusion of the broadest possible sample of healthy and risky behaviors. The additional items were selected from widely used health risk behavior surveys in the public domain: Behavioral Risk Factor Questionnaire (BRFQ; Centers for Disease Control and Prevention, 1993, Health Risk Questionnaire, (Institute for Quality Health [IQH], 1992), and the 1979 National Survey of Personal Health Practices and Health Consequences (NSPHPC; Golden, 1982). The expanded version was used in the psychometric evaluation (Kulbok et al., 1999).

DESCRIPTION OF THE MHBI

The MHBI is a structured, self-administered questionnaire consisting of 57 health-oriented and/or risk-avoidance behaviors in seven sections or scales: Diet (13 items), Substance Use (10 items), Safety (9 items), Check-up (9 items), Social (6 items), Stress (6 items), and Exercise (4 items). (Two questions in the check-up subscale were gender specific: #32 breast self-examination [females only] and #44 testicular self-examination [males only]). These items must be recoded to form one self-examination variable.) Item statements assess the current "relative" frequency of behaviors, from 1 (*never*) to 5 (*always*). The questionnaire stem "How often do you . . ." is followed by items such as "limit fat in your diet," "use drugs to get high," "check the condition of equipment (household, recreational, automotive) regularly" or "exercise vigorously for at least 20 minutes three times a week." To ensure reliability and minimize response set bias, items are worded positively or negatively, similar or inverse questions are asked about selected behaviors where appropriate, and the items are in random order. (See Appendix 1 for a complete copy of the MHBI.)

ADMINISTRATION AND SCORING OF THE MHBI

The general procedure for scoring the MHBI is such that each item is scored from 1 to 5. For items describing a positive health behavior, a score of 1 indicates less frequent behavior and a score of 5 more frequent behavior. Behavioral items, which are worded negatively, implying risky behavior, are recoded accordingly before scoring. (See Appendix 2 for scoring instructions for the MHBI. Asterisks are used to indicate the nine specific items that require reversed scoring.) Item scores are summed for each scale. Scale ranges are as follows: Dietary behaviors (13–65), Substance use/avoidance behaviors (10–50), Safety behaviors (9–45), Check-up behaviors (9–45), Social behaviors (6–30), Stress-related behaviors (6–30), and Exercise behaviors (4–20). Higher scores on the MHBI scales indicate more frequent positive health behavior. The MHBI was not designed for use as a one-dimensional measure or total score.

RELIABILITY AND VALIDITY EVIDENCE

To evaluate the psychometric properties of the MHBI, a convenience sample of 1,077 undergraduate college students completed questionnaires in the classroom or returned them in university mail. This large sample size is recommended to ensure that factors are not simply effects of sampling error (Nunnally & Bernstein, 1994). The mean age of the sample was 20.5 years. Sixty percent were female; 72% were of Caucasian descent, 16% were African American, and the remaining 14% were of Hispanic, Asian, and "other" ethnic origin.

Construct Validity

Descriptive statistics were examined to ensure variability and to satisfy statistical assumptions. Two variables with marked lack of variability were eliminated from all subsequent analyses ("Never used a water pick" and "Never smoked in bed.") Analysis of missing data revealed problems with the five sexual activity variables. Twenty percent of the sample indicated they were not sexually active and did not answer these questions; therefore, the sexual activity variables were eliminated from the analysis. Gender-specific variables such as breast and testicular self-examination were modified to create one self-examination variable. However, there was no equivalent variable for "Pap smear" in the male sample, and that variable was eliminated. Therefore, 116 variables were included in the factor analysis.

Exploratory factor analysis reduced the 116 variables a reasonable set of factors. In this study, .40 was the cutoff value because it provided interpretability of the data (Johnson & Wichern, 1992; Smyth & Yarandi, 1996). The principal component 7-factor solution accounted for a total of 32% of the variance. Varimax and oblique rotations were compared to test the proposition that there are multiple, uncorrelated health behavior dimensions. The factor structure and loadings were strikingly similar for the two methods. The 21 interfactor correlations from the oblique factor rotation were weak, ranging from .02 to .30; therefore, the principal component varimax procedure was used for the final solution. The stability of the 7-factor varimax solution was further evaluated by examining the factor structure and loadings from maximum likelihood factor analysis on the total sample and principal component factor analysis on a split-half sample. These procedures revealed equivalent 7-factor solutions.

Labels for the resulting 7-factor behavior scales were derived from variables with the highest factor loadings. One variable ("Seek health care as needed") had similar loadings on two factors (Checkup: 0.42 and Social: 0.38) and was deleted from the final inventory. Although interpretable 7-factor solution was achieved with 116 variables, the proportion of sample variance explained was improved by factoring the 61 items with factor loadings of 0.40 or greater. Factor analysis of these items confirmed the original 7-factor solution (i.e., the same items loaded on the same factors) and the proportion of variance explained was 45%.

Parallel Item Assessment

There is no other single instrument that measures the breadth of health behaviors included in the MHBI. Therefore, 49 open-ended or multiple response items reporting "specific" frequency of behaviors were included in a Health and Risk Behavior section of the study instrument. Selected questions were "On average, how many hours of sleep do you get in a 24-hour period?" and "In the past 2 weeks, how many days did you drink any alcoholic beverages?" These parallel assessment items were extracted primarily from the IQH, BRFQ, and the NSPHPC to assess validity. Pearson correlation coefficients were computed for pairs of parallel items; all correlation coefficients were greater than .6.

Reliability Analysis

Cronbach's alphas were computed to evaluate the internal consistency of each of the seven health behavior scales of the MHBI (61 items) using the standard of .70 (Nunnally, 1978). Coefficient alphas for the scales ranged from $r = .74$ to $r = .88$. The item-to-total correlations for the seven scales were all above the accepted level of .30 (Nunnally, 1978). Interitem correlations and alpha if an item is deleted were also examined to assess redundancy of items and whether alphas for each scale can be improved. The highest interitem correlation was .72 (factor 1: eat red meat twice a week and eat red meat 1 serving per day). Strickland (1996) suggested that it is difficult to assess items to be truly redundant, unless their correlation with each other is .90 or greater. Final decisions to retain or reject items for the MHBI were based on the results of factor analysis, content validity ratings, and internal consistency analysis. Four items were deleted from the MHBI; the final version includes 7 factor-based scales and 57 items.

CONCLUSION AND RECOMMENDATIONS

Factor analysis of 116 health risk behaviors produced a new health promotion behavior inventory, the MHBI with 57 items and 7 behavior scales. It is important to note that this is the only study that examined such a broad range of health and risk behaviors in young people. The final 7 factor solution with 57 items accounted for 45% of the variance, which exceeds the range of 30% to 41% variance accounted for by others (Aaro, Laberg, & Wold, 1999; Kulbok et al., 1988; Nutbeam, Aaro, & Wold, 1991). Each factor-based scale of the MHBI represents a different dimension of health promotion behavior. The MHBI is not designed for use as a summative scale; rather, the factor-based scales can be used in investigations of antecedents, correlates, or outcomes of different health behavior dimensions. Further evaluation is warranted to assess test-retest reliability and concurrent validity using related instruments with established reliability and validity. In addition, multivariate analysis is needed to examine the stability of relationships within and between different health behavior factors in subgroups defined by age, gender, and race.

The factors identified in this study of college students produced similarities and differences from the behavioral factors in earlier work with adolescents. Although this study used the broadest set of health behaviors, several important behaviors did not have significant factor loadings, for example, using seat belts, eating from "basic" food groups, maintaining desirable weight within limits, avoiding tobacco products, scheduling regular dental checkups, washing hands (after using bathroom), practicing safety rules (when walking or biking), and practicing relaxation or meditation. This study lends support to the assumption that health behaviors of adolescents and college students may be different from adults and may require age-appropriate measurement instruments, such as the one described in this chapter. Clearly, replication of this work with other subgroups of adolescents and young adults is essential to confirm the multiple dimensions of health behavior.

This study is limited by convenience sampling and by the fact that the findings reflect behaviors for young people who are in college. Noncollege students of the same age may have different health behaviors; therefore, health behaviors of young people not enrolled in college need to be examined. The exclusion of the sexual behavior variables from the construct validity assessment is another limitation. In a larger sample of sexually active young people, sexual behavior may emerge as a separate factor. Increasing attention must be focused on the relationship between the prevalence of unsafe sexual behaviors of adolescents and the increase in young adults who are HIV-infected in their 20s (National Community AIDS Partnership, 1993).

The ultimate contribution of this research is the identification of a new measure of health behaviors for an older adolescent and young adult population. This measure is unique in that it includes a broad range of behaviors, measures behavior alone, and is not cluttered by other variables, such as knowledge and perceptions. Behavioral research often focuses on the behavior as an outcome, influenced by knowledge and perceptions, which are targeted for intervention. For a measure to be effective and not introduce collinearity into such outcome research, it must be behavior-specific. The MHBI is such a measure. Future studies with this measure are planned to assess its reliability and validity with subgroups of young people. Once this is achieved, nursing interventions can be tailored for young people to increase positive health outcomes.

REFERENCES

Aaro, L. E., Laberg, J. C., & Wold, B. (1995). Health behavior among adolescents: toward a hypothesis of two dimensions. *Health Education Research, 10*(1), 83–93.

Campbell-Grossman, C., Pozehl, B., & Zimmerman, L. (1996). Nursing students' evaluation of classroom teaching: Development and testing of an instrument. *Journal of Nursing Measurement, 4,* 49–57.

Centers for Disease Control and Prevention. (1993). *1993 Behavioral Risk Factor Questionnaire.* Atlanta: Author.

Donovan, J. E., Jessor, R., & Costa, F. (1993). Structure of health-related behavior in adolescence: A latent-variable approach. *Journal of Health and Social Behavior, 34*(4), 346–362.

Elliott, D. (1993). Health-enhancing and health-compromising lifestyles. In S. G. Millstein, A. C. Petersen, & E. O. Nightengale, (Eds.), *Promoting the health of adolescents: New directions for the twenty-first century* (pp. 119–145). New York: Oxford University Press.

Golden, P. (1982). *Public use data tape documentation; Wave I and Wave II of the National Survey of Personal Health Practices and Consequences, 1979–1980.* Hyattsville, MD: U. S. Department of Health and Human Services, Public Health Service.

Institute for Quality Health. (1992). *Health Risk Questionnaire.* Charlottesville: University of Virginia.

Johnson, R. A., & Wichern, D. W. (1992). *Applied multivariate statistical analysis* (3rd ed.). Englewood Cliffs, NJ: Prentice Hall.

Kulbok, P. (1983). A concept analysis of preventive health behavior. In P. L. Chinn (Ed.), *Advances in nursing theory development* (pp. 125–151). Rockville, MD: Aspen Systems Corp.

Kulbok, P. (1985a). Social resources, health resources, and preventive health behavior: Patterns and predictions. *Public Health Nursing, 2,* 67–81.

Kulbok, P. (1985b, November). *The resource model: Toward a theory of health promotion.* Paper presented at the American Public Health Association annual meeting, Washington, DC.

Kulbok, P. A., & Baldwin, J. (1992). From preventive health behavior to health promotion: Advancing a positive construct of health. *Advances in Nursing Science, 14*(4), 50–64.

Kulbok, P., Baldwin, J., Cox, C. L., & Duffy, R. (1997). Advancing discourse in health promotion: Beyond mainstream thinking. *Advances in Nursing Science, 20*(1), 12–20.

Kulbok, P. A., Carter, K., Baldwin, J., Gilmartin, M, & Kirkwood, B. (1999). The multidimensional health behavior inventory. *Journal of Nursing Measurement, 7,* 177–195.

Kulbok, P., Cary, A. & Seifert, R. (1991, October). *Health promotion: The triad of knowledge, perceptions, and behavior.* Paper presented at the meeting of the Council of Nurse Researchers, Los Angeles.

Kulbok, P., Earls, F., & Montgomery, A. (1988). Lifestyle and patterns of health and social behavior in high-risk adolescents. *Advances in Nursing Science, 11*(2), 22–35.

Kulbok, P., Earls, F., Robins, L., & Jung, K. (1985, November). *Determinants of substance abuse behavior.* Paper presented at the meeting of the American Public Health Association, Washington, DC.

Kulbok, P., Earls, F., Robins, L., Stiffman, & Jung, K. (1985, December). *Factors associated with adolescent substance abuse behavior.* Poster presented at the meeting of the Council of Nurse Researchers, San Diego, CA.

Kurtenbach, S. (1992). *Patterns of health behavior in adolescents.* Masters' thesis, University of Illinois at Chicago.

National Community AIDS Partnership. (1993). *A generation at risk: A background report on HIV prevention and youth.* Washington, DC: Author.

Nunnally, J. (1978). *Psychometric theory* (2nd ed.). New York: McGraw-Hill.

Nunnally, J., & Bernstein, I. (1994). *Psychometric theory* (3rd ed.). New York: McGraw-Hill.

Nutbeam, D., Aaro, L., & Wold, B. (1991). The lifestyle concept and health education with young people: Results from a WHO international survey. *World Health Statistics Quarterly, 44,* 55–61.

Smyth, K., & Yarandi, H. N. (1996). Factor analysis of the ways of coping questionnaire for African American women. *Nursing Research, 45,* 25–29.

Strickland, O. L. (1996). Editorial: Internal consistency analysis: Making the most of what you've got [Editorial]. *Journal of Nursing Measurement, 4,* 3–4.

Zimmerman, L., & Westfall, J. (1985). The development and validation of a scale measuring effective clinical teaching behaviors. *Journal of Nursing Education, 27,* 274–277.

APPENDIX 1: MULTIDIMENSIONAL HEALTH BEHAVIOR INVENTORY

Directions: The following statements describe a broad range of health-related actions or behaviors that you may or may not do. Read each behavior statement and circle the number following each statement that tells how often you do this behavior: 1 = NEVER, 2 = RARELY, 3 = SOMETIMES, 4 = OFTEN, 5 = ALWAYS.

How Often Do You:	Never	Rarely	Sometimes	Often	Always
1. Take time for relaxation every day	1	2	3	4	5
2. Limit red meat in your diet every day.	1	2	3	4	5
3. Plan for home fire escape	1	2	3	4	5
4. Limit fat in your diet every day.	1	2	3	4	5
5. Check your home for safety.	1	2	3	4	5
6. Eat red meat more than two times a week.	1	2	3	4	5
7. Eat fewer calories to lose weight.	1	2	3	4	5
8. Use biodegradable cleaning products.	1	2	3	4	5
9. Ask for help from friends when you are in need.	1	2	3	4	5
10. Avoid being exposed to second hand smoke (someone else smoking at home or at work).	1	2	3	4	5
11. Eat at least one serving or more of red meat on most days (include beef, pork, ham, bacon, lamb, liver, and lunch meat not made from poultry).	1	2	3	4	5
12. Use drugs to get high or to feel better.	1	2	3	4	5
13. Test home smoke detector every month.	1	2	3	4	5
14. Recycle newspaper, glass, and/or other products.	1	2	3	4	5
15. Discuss problems/concerns with someone close to you.	1	2	3	4	5
16. Limit sugar in your diet every day.	1	2	3	4	5
17. Take part in social groups, functions, or classes.	1	2	3	4	5

How Often Do You:	Never	Rarely	Sometimes	Often	Always
18. Eat non-fat or low-fat dairy products.	1	2	3	4	5
19. Do something good for yourself every day.	1	2	3	4	5
20. Choose foods with whole grains every day, for example, whole wheat bread instead of white, brown rice instead of white, etc.	1	2	3	4	5
21. Check your cholesterol level at least once a year.	1	2	3	4	5
22. Seek health information.	1	2	3	4	5
23. Get adequate sleep every day.	1	2	3	4	5
24. Check your blood pressure at least twice a year.	1	2	3	4	5
25. Read food and medicine labels before purchasing or consuming the product.	1	2	3	4	5
26. Question your health care provider or seek a second opinion.	1	2	3	4	5
27. Maintain a first aid kit.	1	2	3	4	5
28. Get 7–8 hours sleep every day.	1	2	3	4	5
29. Praise people easily.	1	2	3	4	5
30. Spend time with close friends.	1	2	3	4	5
31. Participate in recreational physical activities as walking, biking, dancing or sports regularly at least twice a week.	1	2	3	4	5
32. Perform monthly self breast exam. [Answer if female only.]	1	2	3	4	5
33. Limit salt in your diet every day.	1	2	3	4	5
34. Smoke cigarettes every day.	1	2	3	4	5
35. Drink 5 or more alcoholic beverages (beer, wine, wine coolers, or hard liquor) on one occasion.	1	2	3	4	5
36. Check condition of equipment (household, recreational, automotive) regularly.	1	2	3	4	5
37. Limit intake of "sweets" in your diet.	1	2	3	4	5

How Often Do You:	Never	Rarely	Sometimes	Often	Always
38. Do stretching exercises every day.	1	2	3	4	5
39. Fix things as needed.	1	2	3	4	5
40. Obtain a regular health check-up when you are not sick.	1	2	3	4	5
41. Avoid using tobacco products (cigarettes, cigars, pipe chewing tobacco, or snuff).	1	2	3	4	5
42. Control stress in your life.	1	2	3	4	5
43. Exercise vigorously for at least 20 minutes 3 times a week.	1	2	3	4	5
44. Perform monthly self testicular exam. [Answer if male only.]	1	2	3	4	5
45. Keep daily stress levels low.	1	2	3	4	5
46. Avoid drinking and driving.	1	2	3	4	5
47. Increase your physical activity to lose weight.	1	2	3	4	5
48. Run, jog, or swim for exercise at least 3 times per week.	1	2	3	4	5
49. Drink one or more alcoholic beverages (beer, wine, wine coolers, or hard liquor) every day.	1	2	3	4	5
50. Use touch appropriately (hold someone's hand or give someone a hug).	1	2	3	4	5
51. Discuss health concerns with health resource person.	1	2	3	4	5
52. Report unusual or persistent symptoms to a health care provider.	1	2	3	4	5
53. Drink alcohol and take medications at the same time.	1	2	3	4	5
54. Limit your intake of alcoholic beverages (beer, wine, wine coolers, or hard liquor).	1	2	3	4	5
55. Keep emergency numbers by the telephone (poison control, rescue squad, fire department).	1	2	3	4	5

How Often Do You:	Never	Rarely	Sometimes	Often	Always
56. Participate in health care programs (health education, health fair, screening).	1	2	3	4	5
57. Eat at least one or more servings of the following items every day: chips, candy bars, cake, doughnuts, pastries, muffins, cookies, ice cream, pudding, chocolate.	1	2	3	4	5
58. Drink alcohol and drive.	1	2	3	4	5

APPENDIX 2: MULTIDIMENSIONAL HEALTH BEHAVIOR INVENTORY

Scoring Instructions

The MHBI is a structured, self-administered questionnaire. Items are scored from 1 to 5:

$$1 = \text{Never}$$
$$2 = \text{Rarely}$$
$$3 = \text{Sometimes}$$
$$4 = \text{Often}$$
$$5 = \text{Always}$$

For items describing a positive health behavior, a score of 1 indicates less frequent behavior and a score of 5 indicates more frequent behavior. Behavioral items, which are worded negatively implying risky behavior, are recoded before scoring. Higher scores on the MHBI indicate more frequent positive health behavior. The MHBI is designed to assess separate dimensions of health-risk behavior or behavior scales. The MHBI is NOT designed for use as a total score.

*Please note the nine questions, that were worded negatively in the questionnaire are reversed for correct scoring in the subscales below.

	Never	Rarely	Sometimes	Often	Always
Diet (13 items)					
4. Limit fat in diet	1	2	3	4	5
2. Limit red meat	1	2	3	4	5
6. *Eat red meat 2X week	5	4	3	2	1
11. *Red meat 1 serving/day	5	4	3	2	1
18. Eat nonfat dairy	1	2	3	4	5
7. Limit calorie intake	1	2	3	4	5
16. Limit sugar intake	1	2	3	4	5
37. Limit sweets in diet	1	2	3	4	5
57. *Eat one serving junk food	5	4	3	2	1
47. Exercise to lose weight	1	2	3	4	5
33. Limit salt intake	1	2	3	4	5
20. Eat whole grain foods	1	2	3	4	5
25. Read food labels	1	2	3	4	5
Substance Use (10 items)					
35. *5/more alcoholic drinks	5	4	3	2	1
54. Limit alcoholic intake	1	2	3	4	5
12. *Use drugs to get high	5	4	3	2	1
49. *Drink alcohol daily	5	4	3	2	1

	Never	Rarely	Sometimes	Often	Always
10. Avoid second-hand smoke	1	2	3	4	5
34. *Smoke cigarettes daily	5	4	3	2	1
53. *Drink & take medication	5	4	3	2	1
58. *Drink & drive	5	4	3	2	1
46. Avoid drinking & driving.	1	2	3	4	5
41. Avoid using tobacco products	1	2	3	4	5

Safety/Environment (9 items)

36. Check equipment	1	2	3	4	5
13. Check fire detector	1	2	3	4	5
27. Maintain first-aid kit	1	2	3	4	5
39. Fix thinks as needed	1	2	3	4	5
8. Use biodegradable products	1	2	3	4	5
5. Check home for safety	1	2	3	4	5
55. Emergency phone numbers	1	2	3	4	5
3. Plan home fire escape	1	2	3	4	5
14. Recycle	1	2	3	4	5

Checkup (9 items)**

51. Discuss health concerns	1	2	3	4	5
40. Obtain regular checkup	1	2	3	4	5
22. Seek health information	1	2	3	4	5
26. Seek second opinion	1	2	3	4	5
52. Report persistent symptoms	1	2	3	4	5
56. Seek health education	1	2	3	4	5
24. Check blood pressure	1	2	3	4	5
32. **Perform monthly BSE	1	2	3	4	5
44. **Perform monthly TSE	1	2	3	4	5
21. Check cholesterol level	1	2	3	4	5

Social (6 items)

30. Spend time with friends	1	2	3	4	5
15. Discuss problems with friends	1	2	3	4	5
9. Ask a friend for help	1	2	3	4	5
17. Participate in social activities	1	2	3	4	5
50. Use touch appropriately	1	2	3	4	5
29. Praise people easily	1	2	3	4	5

Stress/Rest (6 items)

42. Control stress in your life	1	2	3	4	5

	Never	Rarely	Sometimes	Often	Always
45. Keep daily stress levels low	1	2	3	4	5
23. Get adequate sleep every day	1	2	3	4	5
28. Sleep 7–8 hours a day	1	2	3	4	5
19. Do something good for yourself.	1	2	3	4	5
1. Take time to relax every day.	1	2	3	4	5
Exercise (4 items)					
43. Exercise vigorously.	1	2	3	4	5
48. Aerobic activities/exercise	1	2	3	4	5
31. Enjoy recreational activities.	1	2	3	4	5
38. Stretch muscles	1	2	3	4	5

19

The Compliance Questionnaire

Gail A. Hilbert-McAllister

This chapter discusses the Compliance Questionnaire (CQ), a measure of patient compliance with therapeutic regimens.

PURPOSE

The purpose of this chapter is to examine a number of issues related to the measurement of compliance. These issues will be addressed in relation to an investigation of compliance of myocardial infarction (MI) patients (Hilbert, 1983). The instrument used in this study was a self-report questionnaire with a Likert-type scale. Content validity and interrater reliability were obtained. Triangulation of data from three different sources (participant, spouse, and investigator) provided further support for the validity of the tool.

CONCEPTUAL FRAMEWORK

A commonly used definition of *compliance* is that of Sackett (1976): "the extent to which the patient's behavior coincides with the clinical prescription" (p. 1). As early as 1974 there was concern about the connotations of the word *compliance,* which suggests a dictatorial process in which the clinician does not involve the patient. At that time, an interdisciplinary group at the Workshop/Symposium on Compliance with Therapeutic Regimens at McMaster University expanded the definition of *compliance* to "the extent to which the patient's behavior coincides with the clinical prescription regardless of how the latter was generated" (Sackett, 1976, p. 1). The authors went on to say that the term *compliance* describes the extent to which the patient yields to health instructions and advice "whether declared by an autocratic, authoritarian clinician or developed as a consensual regimen through negotiation between a health professional and a citizen" (p. 2).

In 1979, an interdisciplinary group (Barofsky, Sugarbaker, & Mills) described a social control continuum with three points: compliance, adherence, and therapeutic alliance. They stated that any patient–provider relationship has had or does have elements of all three types of relationships. *Compliance* describes a standard external to both parties. *Adherence* is a more appropriate term when both patient and provider expect a particular pattern of behavior, and it implies less social control as a result of interaction between the two. Therapeutic alliance implies negotiations that have resulted in acceptance of the regimen. A therapeutic alliance should develop over time if the patient is able to negotiate with the health care provider and assume responsibility for self-care.

By 1982, a number of articles by nurses addressed the issue of whether *compliance* and *noncompliance* were appropriate terms for nursing. Dracup and Meleis (1982) described these terms using an interactionist approach. They stated that there is a false assumption underlying the medical model that describes noncompliance in terms of the characteristics of the patient alone, rather than focusing on characteristics of both patient and health professional and on the interaction between them.

An issue of *Nursing Clinics of North America* addressed the topic of patient compliance in September 1982. Conway-Rutkowski (1982), editor of that issue, noted the paucity of research about the negotiation process in which the nurse and patient participate to select an appropriate therapeutic plan. In that same issue, Moughton (1982) suggested the use of the term *therapeutic alliance* and advocated involving the patient in the nursing care plan.

Wuest (1993) questioned the appropriateness of noncompliance as a nursing diagnosis. She reviewed the nursing literature, critiquing studies of noncompliance. She concluded that the Health Belief Model, frequently a theoretical framework for research, arises from the medical model and recommended examining quality of life in relation to compliance. She also concluded that the term *noncompliance* be eliminated from nursing taxonomy to indicate a willingness to seek new approaches to a very complex concern.

The development of the Compliance Questionnaire (CQ) was initiated in 1979, when the issue of the compliance versus the therapeutic alliance was not considered by the researcher in the choice of a theoretical definition. The definition chosen was that previously quoted from Sackett (1976, p. 1): "the extent to which the patient's behavior coincides with the clinical prescription." The prescription with which the participant was complying was that of the health team, as recalled by the participant. During semistructured interviews with the MI patients and their spouses, it became apparent that very little "tailoring of the consensual regimen," a phrase coined by Fink (1976), had taken place.

PROCEDURES FOR DEVELOPMENT AND DESCRIPTION

Prior to development of the instrument, a review of the compliance literature located three studies dealing with compliance of MI patients. Johnson (1974) interviewed 225 married males under 75 years of age who had experienced a first MI. Marston (1969) conducted interviews of 28 male MI patients between the ages of 44 and 64. Bille (1975) did telephone interviews of 24 males ages 32 to 75.

Johnson (1974) adapted an instrument used by Davis (cited in Marston, 1969). (Johnson developed the instrument in 1964, but it was not published until 1974, thus the seeming discrepancy in the dates.) Johnson's instrument included eight areas of recommendations: medications, diet, physical activity, smoking, alcohol use, stress, exercise, and sexual intercourse. Participants were asked to describe the physician's recommendations in each area and any difficulties encountered, and to rate themselves as to how well they had been able to follow each recommendation. The rating categories were "all of the time," "most of the time," "less than half of the time," and "very little or not at all."

Marston (1969) adapted Johnson's unpublished instrument. She added the categories of weight loss and work to this questionnaire and eliminated sexual intercourse. She used the same format, in terms of questioning for additional information and a similar rating scale, separating out "very little" and "not at all" into two categories. She also added a numerical value, ranging from 4 (*all of the time*) to 0 (*not at all*).

Bille (1975) used the same categories and rating scale as Marston (1969). He conducted telephone interviews and developed guidelines for placing participants in categories when discrepant information was obtained. For example, when participants rated themselves low on medication compliance because they did not take a prn medication, they would be placed in the "all of the time" category.

The present instrument (Hilbert, 1983, 1985a, 1985b) added caffeine use to the 10 categories of compliance used in the instruments described above. The respondent was instructed to recall recommendations made by the health team rather than the physician. This was based on the assumption that nurses, dietitians, and other members of the health care team are involved in instructing MI patients about their therapeutic regimens. The participants were also instructed to limit their recall of how well they had carried out the instructions to the previous week. This was because the researcher was interested in recent compliance and because it was thought that this would allow for more accurate recall. For the present instrument, participants indicated their compliance using the Likert-type scale of Marston (1969), ranging from 4 (*all of the time*) to 0 (*none of the time*).

Content validity of the questionnaire was determined by a panel of three nurses with master of science degrees in nursing who had expertise in the area of coronary rehabilitation. The 11 categories of compliance were also consistent with the information found in the protocol of the teaching plan for one of the cardiac rehabilitation programs from which the participants were obtained (Widemer, 1979). The category of sexual advice was later removed when it was found that none of the 60 participants had been given specific advice in this area. All participants had been told to resume whatever was normal for them or had been given no advice in this area. The final instrument contained the following categories: medication, diet, weight reduction, stress reduction, exercise, physical activity, smoking cessation, alcohol and caffeine use, and work (Hilbert, 1983).

ADMINISTRATION AND SCORING

Although a continuous score allows for more powerful statistical manipulation, some types of compliance are categorical by their nature. For example, receiving an immunization would be categorized into "yes" and "no." Other times a participant may be placed in a category based on the distribution of scores, such as a median split or quartiles. Gordis (1979) recommends using a biologic rationale, such as the level of compliance required to achieve a therapeutic response for dichotomizing patients into compliers and noncompliers. In the absence of such information, it is possible to select an arbitrary level of compliance as adequate.

When there is more than one area of compliance to be measured, it is necessary to decide whether or not to use a composite score. In the present study, it was possible that a participant would have some recommendations that would not apply, for example, the individual who was of normal weight at the time of the MI and thus had no recommendation regarding weight loss. This was handled by having a "not applicable" option. A total compliance score was then derived by totaling the scores for all recommendations that were applicable and dividing by the total possible score, resulting in a percentage score. It was deemed important to use separate areas of compliance, as well as the total score, in hypothesis testing because there was no evidence that the individual scores would be highly intercorrelated.

Another decision regarding the calculation of compliance scores is whether or not to weight scores based on information that may be obtained in addition to the participant's self-report. One possible approach is to weight each item of the regimen according to the importance of that item. Davis (cited in Marston, 1969) developed a composite index based on the physician's actual recommendation, patient's and physician's independent estimates of the degree of compliance, and a weighting factor derived from the physician's evaluation of the relative importance of various components of the regimen.

Another approach to deriving a score would be to examine the degree of change by comparing present behavior with previous behavior for each recommendation. This is based on the assumption that 100% compliance with a particular recommendation may indicate a great deal of change for one patient and little for another. For example, a patient who smoked two packs of cigarettes per day before the MI and then stopped has had to change more than the person who smoked five cigarettes. No study that used this method was located, but it is something that should be considered as a possibility to allow for more meaningful comparative scores.

Still another approach is to consider the amount of difficulty involved in achieving the recommendation. Although for some participants the amount of difficulty may be synonymous with the amount of change, there is no empirical evidence to support this assumption. Difficulty may be considered by looking at the success rate for each recommendation across participants. Those recommendations with low compliance means would be considered more difficult than those with higher mean achievement, thus allowing a weighting formula to be developed. It is also possible to obtain the participants' estimates of the relative difficulty in achieving each recommendation and devise a weighting schema based on that information.

RELIABILITY AND VALIDITY

The study for which the CQ was developed focused on the influence of spouse support on the compliance of 60 male participants ages 38 to 73 who were at least 3 months post-MI. The theoretical framework was based on both the social support and compliance literatures. Spouse support was assumed to be a specific category of social support that has been linked with the ability to cope with stress, as well as being positively related to a variety of health outcomes (House, 1981). Spouse support was defined as the degree to which the spouse of an MI patient engaged in activities directed toward providing her husband with physical assistance, intimate interaction, social participation, material aid, guidance, and feedback (Barrera & Ainlay, 1983).

A decision was made to use self-reports obtained during home interviews for the present study. The interview allowed the investigator to assess the participant's recall of recommendations and discuss any problems encountered in carrying them out. It also allowed the investigator to note discrepancies between self-report and environmental evidence, such as the presence of foods that were not allowed on the participant's diet. It was not assumed that the participant was noncompliant in such cases. However, the investigator was then able to question whether or not the participant usually included such foods in his diet on a regular basis. It was also noted that a number of participants smoked during the interview, verifying their noncompliance in that area.

In a manner similar to the husband, the wife was asked to describe her understanding of her husband's recommendations and any difficulties he encountered in carrying them out. She then rated her perceptions of her husband's compliance in each area for the previous week. The husband and wife were interviewed separately, and all interviews were tape-recorded.

The investigator also determined a judged compliance score, which was based on her detection of discrepancies within the self-reports. For example, if a participant had given himself a 4 (*all of the time*) rating but made statements about not complying all of the time—missing doses of medication, drinking caffeinated coffee when instructed not to do so, exceeding the recommended amounts of alcohol, eating foods not allowed on a low-sodium or modified-fat diet, engaging in activities forbidden by the doctor, exceeding the calorie limit, smoking or not meeting the exercise recommendations—the judged score was lower than the participant's self reported score.

If a participant rated himself lower than would be expected—for example, had rated himself low on medication compliance, but the medication was related to need and did not have to be taken everyday, or he was allowed some caffeine or alcohol and had not exceeded the limit—the judged score was higher than the self-report score. The judged compliance score for each participant and each category might be the same as the self-report, higher, or lower.

Interrater reliability was determined by having a second rater listen to the tapes and record compliance scores for the first five interviews and every 10th interview thereafter. The interrater reliability was .96 for both the self-reported compliance scores and the wife's rating and .84 for the judged compliance scores.

The judged ratings and the self-reported ratings were correlated significantly for all 10 aspects of the regimen, ranging from .531 to .994 ($p <$ .001). Husbands and wives also had significantly correlated ratings (from .297 to .972) at the .001 level, with the exception of alcohol use (.419 at $p < .05$), physical activity (.101), and stress reduction (.247), which were not significantly correlated. These findings from triangulation of data lent further support to the validity and reliability of the tool.

The investigator found that participants were able to admit to considerable noncompliance. For example, a number of participants rated themselves low for diet, weight loss, and stress reduction. As might be expected, weight reduction was a difficult area in which to achieve compliance, with participants reporting a mean compliance of 64%, based on the ratio of the reported scores to the highest possible score. Of the 33 participants who were smoking at the time of the Ml, 6 were still smoking and did so during the interviews.

It was concluded that participants rate themselves accurately in direct interviews conducted by an investigator who has established rapport and communicates concern. An introductory comment about understanding how difficult it is to comply and that most patients are not completely compliant sets the right atmosphere.

The interview format allows the investigator to find out the participants' recall of recommendations, thus stimulating their memories. Questions can focus on prescriptions, diet pamphlets, and teaching programs, as well as the day-to-day manner in which the participant attempts to carry out the recommendations. The interview format also allows for gentle probing if there are any discrepancies, for example, "Think back to the past week and tell me how many doses of your medication you think you missed" or "What do you do about your diet if you are eating in a restaurant?"

Although no method of assessing compliance is ideal, and the optimal method will vary with the type of compliance being assessed, interview methods incorporating the previous suggestions should allow researchers to place greater confidence in the validity of the data obtained.

Since 1993, the CQ has been used in numerous unpublished theses and dissertations (Scott, 1997; Segreti, 1992). A review of the literature reveals that the CQ is useful in two ways. First, it provides a methodology for measuring compliance for several medical conditions that require lifestyle change. For example, Evangelista, Berg, and Dracup (2001) used a modified version of the CQ that addressed the regimen issues common to patients with heart failure, as did Scott (1997) who adapted the CQ for use with hemodialysis patients.

Second, the CQ validates the use of self-report as a means of obtaining data on compliance. Numerous articles have cited Hilbert (1985a) to support the validity of compliance measures (Dew, Roth, Thompson, Kormos, & Griffith, 1996; Evangelista et al., 2001; Wong, Wong, Nolde, & Yabsley (1990). The present study, reported above, showed high intercorrelations among self-report, spouse report, and the judged score. Also, the face-to-face interview format appears to allow for participants to admit to considerable compliance, thus appearing to mitigate against the social desirability aspect of self-report scales.

CONCLUSIONS AND RECOMMENDATIONS

This chapter described the development of an instrument that measures compliance for 10 aspects of the MI regimen. Researchers are urged to give careful consideration to decisions relating to their choice of both theoretical and operational definitions of compliance.

Questions to be considered include the following:

1. Is the theoretical definition congruent with the nursing conceptual framework?
2. With whose prescriptions is the participant complying?
3. How will compliance scores be calculated for maximum utility in terms of comparability with other participants and studies and for statistical analysis?
4. Should self-report scores be used, or are more objective means available?
5. How can one protect noncompliant participants from loss of confidentiality while at the same time ensuring that they will not endanger their health?

In regard to the calculation of compliance scores, when there are a number of items in the therapeutic plan, scores should be calculated for each aspect as well as for the total plan. Scores based on weighted composites of a number of factors have been suggested, such as importance of each item, amount of change required, and difficulty in achieving each recommendation. Consideration of these factors may result in a more valid measurement of compliance.

The issue of the accuracy of self-reported compliance has been discussed. The study of compliance of MI patients suggested that participants do admit to noncompliance if the investigator establishes rapport and communicates acceptance of less than perfect compliance. Home interviews using gentle probing will help the participant recall deviations from the prescribed regimen.

Finally, an instrument for measuring compliance of MI patients has been described. Content validity and interrater reliability have been assessed for this instrument. Concurrent ratings by the researcher and the subject's spouse yielded further evidence of the validity of the instrument.

REFERENCES

Barofsky, I., Sugarbaker, P H., & Mills, M. E. (1979). Compliance and quality of life assessment. In J. Cohen (Ed), *New directions in patient compliance* (pp. 59–74). Lexington, MA: D. C. Heath.

Barrera, M., & Ainlay, S. L. (1983). The structure of social support: A conceptual and empirical analysis. *Journal of Community Psychology 11,* 133–143.

Bille, D. A. (1975). *Structured vs. unstructured teaching format and body image, compliance with post-hospitalization prescriptions and knowledge about life following heart attack.* Unpublished doctoral dissertation, University of Wisconsin, Madison.

Conway-Rutkowsky, B. (1982). Foreword to symposium on patient compliance. *Nursing Clinics of North America, 17,* 440–450.

Dew, M. A., Roth, L. H., Thompson, M. E., Kormos, R. L., & Griffith, B. P. (1996). Medical compliance and its predictors in the first year after heart transplantation. *Journal of Heart Lung Transplant, 15,* 631–645.

Dracup, K. A., & Meleis, A. I. (1982). Compliance: An interactionist approach. *Nursing Research, 21,* 37–42.

Evangelista, L. S., Berg, J., & Dracup, K. (2001). Relationship between psychosocial variables and compliance in patients with heart failure. *Heart and Lung, 30,* 294–301.

Fink, D. L. (1976). Tailoring the consensual regimen. In D. L. Sackett & R. B. Haynes (Eds.), *Compliance with therapeutic regimens* (pp. 110–118). Baltimore, MD: Johns Hopkins University Press.

Gordis, K. (1979). Conceptual and methodologic problems in measuring patient compliance. In R. B. Haynes, D. W. Taylor, & D. L. Sackett (Eds.), *Compliance in health care* (pp. 23–45). Baltimore: Johns Hopkins University Press.

Hilbert, G. K. (1983). *The relationship between spouse support and compliance of the myocardial infarction patients.* Unpublished doctoral dissertation, University of Pennsylvania, Philadelphia.

Hilbert, G. (1985a). On the accuracy of self reported measures of compliance. *Nursing Research, 34,* 319–320.

Hilbert, G. (1985b). Spouse support and myocardial infarction patient compliance. *Nursing Research, 34,* 217–220.

Hilbert, G. (1988). The measurement of compliance as a nursing outcome. In C. F. Waltz & O. L. Strickland (Eds.), *Measurement of nursing outcomes* (pp. 80–107). New York: Springer Publishing Co.

House, J. S. (1981). *Work, stress and social support.* Reading, MA: Addison-Wesley.

Johnson, W. L. (1974). *Adjustment to the crisis of coronary heart disease.* New York: National League for Nursing.

Marston, M. V. (1969). *Compliance with medical regimens as a form of risk-taking in patients with myocardial infarctions.* Unpublished doctoral dissertation, Boston University, Boston.

Moughton, M. (1982). The patient—a partner in the health care process. *Nursing Clinics of North America, 17,* 3.

Sackett, D. L. (1976). Introduction. In D. L. Sackett & R. B. Haynes (Eds.). *Compliance with therapeutic regimens* (pp. 1–6). Baltimore, MD: Johns Hopkins University Press.

Scott, S. B. (1997). *Exploration of factors that impact mode of death in the hemodialysis patient.* Unpublished doctoral dissertation, Kent State University, Kent, Ohio.

Segreti, A. (1992). *Relationship of functional social support to psychological adjustment and treatment compliance following initial myocardial infarction.*

Unpublished doctoral dissertation, Hofstra University, Hempstead, New York.

Widemer, N. (1979). *Inpatient cardiac education.* Philadelphia: Albert Einstein Medical Center, Daroff Division.

Wong, J., Wong, S., Nolde, T. & Yabsley, R. H. (1990). Effects of an experimental program on post-hospital adjustment of early discharged patients. *International Journal of Nursing Studies, 27,* 7–20.

Wuest, J. (1993). Removing the shackles: A feminist critique of non-compliance. *Nursing Outlook, 41,* 217–224.

APPENDIX: COMPLIANCE QUESTIONNAIRE

Patient

Instructions: The questions you will be asked have to do with recommendations you have been told to follow by the health team (nurses, doctors, physical therapists, dietitians, etc.).

I.   Let's start with **MEDICATIONS**.

   A.   Are you taking medicine of any kind?

   Name   *Dose*   *Frequency*

   1.
   2.
   3.
   4.

   B.   Have you had any difficulty with taking any of these? What kind of difficulty (e.g., remembering, inconvenience, cost, side effects, etc.)?

   C.   For the drugs mentioned: Would you estimate that you have been taking it (in the past week):

   Judged Score

   _____   ___ (4) all of the time
   _____   ___ (3) most of the time
   _____   ___ (2) about half of the time
   _____   ___ (1) very seldom
   _____   ___ (0) none of the time

   D.   Do you think you missed any doses in the past week? How many?

   E.   What has been helpful in regard to your taking the medications as directed?

   What has not been helpful?

II. Let's go to **DIET** other than weight reduction.

   A.   Are you on a diet? What kind?
   B.   Did anyone on the health team (doctor, nurse, dietitian, physical therapist, etc.) make suggestions regarding your eating patterns (e.g., reduce the amount of salt and salty foods, reduce the amount of fat, change the kind of fat, reduce or eliminate certain foods)?

If so, what was recommended? Were you given diet sheet? Have you read books, pamphlets?

C. Who prepares this? Who does the food shopping?

D. Have you had any difficulty with following your dietary recommendations? If so, what kind of difficulty? What about eating out, going to parties, etc.?

E. Would you estimate that you have been able to follow your diet (in the past week):

Judged Score
_____	_____	(4) all of the time
_____	_____	(3) most of the time
_____	_____	(2) about half of the time
_____	_____	(1) very seldom
_____	_____	(0) none of the time

F. What has been helpful for you in regard to carrying out these recommendations?

What has not been helpful?

III. Let's go to **WEIGHT LOSS**.

A. Did anyone on the health team make any recommendations concerning loss of weight?

If so, what were you told?
Loose weight, maintain same weight?

Who made the recommendation?

B. If you were told to lose weight, how much were you told to lose?

C. Which method was recommended?

D. Over how long a period of time were you to have lost this?

E. Have you lost weight, maintained same weight, or gained weight?

F. How much have you lost or gained?

G. Have you had any difficulty in following the recommendations for weight loss?

H. What kind of difficulty?

I. In the past week, how much of the time have you followed the recommendations regarding your weight reduction?

Judged Score
_____   _____ (4) all of the time
_____   _____ (3) most of the time
_____   _____ (2) about half of the time
_____   _____ (1) very seldom
_____   _____ (0) not at all

J. What has been helpful in regard to carrying out these recommendations?
What has not been helpful?

IV. Let's go to **PHYSICAL ACTIVITY**, in terms of activity that could be considered harmful.

A. Did any member of the health team suggest that you limit your activity in any way (e.g., avoiding strenuous activity, avoiding working or exercising in very hot or very cold weather, avoiding isometric exercise, lifting a maximum amount of weight, mowing the lawn, shoveling snow)?

What were you told?

Who made the recommendation?

B. Have you had any difficulty in following these recommendations?

C. What kind of difficulty have you had?

D. Would you estimate that you have been able to follow these recommendations (in the past week):

Judged Score
_____   _____ (4) all of the time
_____   _____ (3) most of the time
_____   _____ (2) about half of the time
_____   _____ (1) very seldom
_____   _____ (0) none of the time

E. What has been helpful in carrying out these recommendations?

F. What has not been helpful?

V. Let's go to **EXERCISE** that could be considered helpful.

A. Did any member of the health team suggest that you engage in an exercise program (daily walks, using an exercise bike, using a treadmill, swimming, etc.)?

What recommendations were made? How often did you go to the rehab program? If done at home, optimal pulse rate.

Who made them?

B. Have you had any difficulty in following these recommendations?

C. What kind of difficulty?

D. Would you estimate that you have been able to follow these recommendations:

Judged Score
_____   _____ (4) all of the time
_____   _____ (3) most of the time
_____   _____ (2) about half of the time
_____   _____ (1) very seldom
_____   _____ (0) none of the time

E. What has been helpful in carrying out these recommendations?

What has not been helpful?

VI. Let's go to **STRESSFUL SITUATIONS**.

A. Did any member of the health team recommend that you try to avoid stressful situations or make changes in your life to better deal with stress when it arises (e.g., set practical goals, lighten your load of responsibility, discuss problems with someone, set aside a time each day for relaxation, etc.)?

Who made the suggestions?

What suggestions were made? Was anything specific said?

B. Have you had any difficulty in following this advice?

C. What kind of difficulty have you had?

D. Would you say that you have been able to avoid stressful situations or deal with stress in specific ways (in the past week):

Judged Score
_____   _____ (4) all of the time
_____   _____ (3) most of the time
_____   _____ (2) about half of the time
_____   _____ (1) very seldom
_____   _____ (0) not at all

E. What has been helpful in carrying out these recommendations?

What has not been helpful?

VII. Let's go to **SMOKING**.

    A.   Did you smoke prior to your illness?

        If yes, how much of each of the following per day?
        ____ cigarettes ____ cigars ____ pipe

    B.   Did anyone of the health team suggest that you cut down or eliminate smoking?

        If so, who made the recommendation?

        Did anyone suggest a method for stopping smoking?

    C.   Have you had any difficulty in following this advice?

    D.   What kind of difficulty have you had?

    E.   How much of the time have you followed these recommendations in the past week:

    Judged Score
        ____   ____ (4) all of the time
        ____   ____(3) most of the time
        ____   ____(2) about half of the time
        ____   ____(1) very seldom
        ____   ____ (0) not at all

    F.   How much do you smoke now?
        ____ cigarettes ____ cigars ____ pipe

    G.   What has been helpful in carrying out these recommendations?

        What has not been helpful?

VIII.   Let's go to **ALCOHOL USE**.

    A.   Did you drink alcoholic beverages before your illness? if yes, how much per week? ____beer ____ wine ____ hard liquor

B. Did anyone on the health team make any recommendations to you about alcohol use?

What were you told?

By whom?

C. Have you had any difficulty in following this advice?

D. What kind of difficulty have you had?

E. How much of the time have you followed these recommendations in the past week?

Judged Score
____   ____ (4) all of the time
____   ____ (3) most of the time
____   ____ (2) about half of the time
____   ____ (1) very seldom
____   ____(0) not at all

F. How much do you now drink per week?
____ beer ____wine ____ hard liquor

G. What has been helpful in regard to following the recommendations about alcohol use?

What has not been helpful?

IX. Let's go to **CAFFEINE INTAKE.**

A. Did you drink beverages containing caffeine, such as coffee, tea, or colas, before your illness?

B. If so, how much per day? ___ coffee ___ tea ___ colas

C. Did anyone on the health team make any recommendations about intake of beverages containing caffeine (coffee, tea, colas)?

Who made the recommendations?

What was recommended?

D. Have you had any difficulty in following these recommendations?

E. If so, what kind of difficulty have you had?

F. How often in the last week would you estimate that you have been following the recommendations about caffeine intake?

Judged Score
_____   _____(4) all of the time
_____   _____(3) most of the time
_____   _____(2) about half of the time
_____   _____(1) very seldom
_____   _____(0) none of the time

G. How much are you now drinking of beverages containing caffeine per day? _____ coffee _____ tea ___ colas

H. What has been helpful in carrying out these recommendations? What has not been helpful?

X. Let's go to **SEXUAL ACTIVITY**

A. Did anyone on the health team make recommendations about sexual activity (positions, relationship to meals and alcoholic beverages, using nitroglycerin, etc.)?

B. What recommendations were made? Who made them?

C. What changes have occurred in your sexual relationship with your wife since your illness?

What are your thoughts about factors that have contributed to these changes?

D. Have you had any difficulties in carrying out the recommendations of the health team about sexual activity? (If recommendations applied to a limited period and no longer apply, skip D and E.)

E. In the past month how much of the time have your carried out the recommendations about sexual activity?

Judged Score
____	____(4) all of the time
____	____(3) most of the time
____	____(2) about half of the time
____	____(1) very seldom
____	____(0) none of the time

F. What has been helpful in adjusting sexually since your illness?

What has not been helpful?

XI. Let's go to **WORK**.

A. What was your occupation before you became ill?

B. Did anyone on the health team suggest any changes be made in regard to your work?

Who made the recommendation?

What was recommended?

C. Have you returned to work? If so:

_____ same job as before
_____ same job but with fewer demands
_____ same job but with shorter hours
____different job ____totally different
____somewhat different ____slightly different

If you are in a different job, what are you now doing?

D. If you have not returned to work, do you plan to return to work?

If yes, how will you decide on a future job?
____ own judgment
____ health team advice
____ other, specify

E. If anyone on the health team made recommendations regarding changes in work, have you had difficulty in following these recommendations?

If yes, what kinds of difficulty?

F. How much of the time are you currently following recommendations in regard to work?

Judged Score
____   ____ (4) all of the time
____   ____ (3) most of the time
____   ____ (2) about half of the time
____   ____ (1) very seldom
____   ____ (0) none of the time

G. What has been helpful in adjusting to the changes you have had to make in regard to work?

What has not been helpful?

20

The Index of Readiness

Julie Fleury and Kim Cameron

This chapter discusses the Index of Readiness, a measure of motivation appraisal of readiness to initiate behavioral change.

PURPOSE

Lifestyle patterns and personal habits remain the leading cause of death and premature disability in industrialized countries (Public Health Service, U. S. Department of Health and Human Services, 1990). Individual risk reduction through the initiation and maintenance of preventive health behaviors, including smoking cessation, hypertensive management, regular physical activity, and dietary modification, has been linked with a reduced morbidity from chronic illness and an enhanced quality of life. Although many physical and behavioral characteristics that increase the risk of developing acute and chronic illnesses have been established, the challenge of promoting sustained lifestyle change to reduce or eliminate risk-producing behaviors has not been met.

Effective health promotion efforts targeting the primary and secondary prevention of illness are guided by relevant theory and theory-based interventions to enhance individual motivation and promote resources for behavioral change. Motivation in health behavior change is conceptualized as a process of intention formation and goal-directed behavior that guides the creation of positive health patterns (Fleury, 1991). An understanding of motivation to initiate behavioral change is considered an essential first step in creating a lasting program of risk modification. However, the appraisal of readiness to initiate health behavior change represents a motivational concept that has not been systematically examined or indexed conceptually. This chapter outlines advances in the development and psychometric testing of the Index of Readiness (Fleury, 1993, 1994), a measure of motivation appraisal of readiness to initiate behavioral change.

CONCEPTUAL BASIS OF THE INDEX OF READINESS

The instrumentation efforts described were based on the wellness motivation theory, which includes an analysis of how people generate goals, imagine opportunities for action, and create and execute strategies of health-relevant behavioral change (Fleury, 1991, 1994, 1996). In the wellness motivation theory, behavioral change is conceptualized as a process of intention formation and goal-directed activity that guides the creation of positive health patterns. The model consists of three dimensions: contextual influences, behavioral change processes, and action.

The initiation and maintenance of behavioral change are thought to occur within, or in interaction with, the person's environment. Contextual influences originate either within the individual or as a part of the individual's environment, including the social, cultural, biological, and physical environment. Contextual influences both shape and are shaped by personal values, goals, expectations, and strategies for action (Ewart, 1991). Such influences may have a significant impact in creating a supportive personal and ecological environment to promote behavioral change processes.

Behavioral change processes reflect the ways in which individuals create and evaluate goals, establish standards for behavioral change, determine behavioral strategies, and regulate and strengthen patterns of behavioral change (Bandura, 1989; Carver & Scheier, 1981; Fleury, 1991, 1996). Behavioral change processes illustrate a fundamental characteristic of individual motivation, the propensity to strive toward new goals and move beyond goals that have been achieved (Fleury, 1991, 1996). Behavioral change processes include self-knowledge, motivation appraisal, and self-regulation.

Self-knowledge is that aspect of the self-concept that reflects motivational needs expressed as individual goals (Markus & Nurius, 1986). Self-knowledge serves to frame and guide the generation of individual goals and behavioral intentions (Bandura, 1986; Fleury, 1991, 1996). As an essential preparatory stage within behavioral change, self-knowledge includes multiple aspects of the self that develop through internal self-evaluation and interpersonal experiences, and reflect values and goals, perceived efficacy, and strategies for guiding and regulating personal behavior (Fleury, 1991; Markus & Wurf, 1987). Individuals select goals that represent not just desired outcomes, but outcomes related to valued representations of the self, or enduring self-definitions (Fleury, 1991; Markus & Nurius, 1986). Self-knowledge also contains cultural meaning, which shapes individual motives and goals (D'Andrade, 1990).

Motivation appraisal is that part of the motivational system that guides intention formation as part of the individual's evaluation of readiness to initiate behavioral change (Fleury, 1991, 1996). Motivation appraisal of readiness to initiate health behavior change occurs through the determination of valued goals; cognitive preparation for action, including the assessment of current behavior, planning, and strategy selection; and the determination of standards for self-monitoring, judgment, and evaluation (Fleury, 1991). Through an assessment of goals and judgments about the means best suited to attain those goals, individuals generate plans and strategies for goal attainment, engage in problem solving, and determine commitment to valued goals (Fleury, 1991, 1996; Gollwitzer, 1987; Nuttin, 1987). Motivation appraisal may be compared with an individually constructed map or model for behavioral change that outlines expected behavior, as well as how behavior might be managed and evaluated (Ewart, 1991; Karoly, 1995).

Self-regulation includes those cognitive, affective, and behavioral strategies through which people attempt to make behavior congruent with valued goals, particularly when goals conflict or change (Ewart, 1991; Bandura, 1986; Karoly, 1995). Acknowledgment of self-regulatory mechanisms is essential because long-term adherence to behavioral change requires strategies for motivating behavioral change and effectively responding to contextual influences. The pursuit and attainment of self-generated goals and the maintenance of self-determined standards for behavior are critical sources of motivation that involve the internal regulation of behavior (Kuhl, 1987). Thus, self-regulation includes the evaluation of response to contextual influences and appraisal of personal efforts at self-management. Action incorporates the individual's response to contextual influences and behavioral change processes. Action specific to health behavior change may be evaluated on a number of levels, including subjective response, objective evaluation, and physiologic or biologic response.

PROCEDURES FOR DEVELOPMENT

The instrumentation efforts described are focused on the operationalization and refinement of the concept of motivation appraisal as a behavioral change process in the initiation of behavioral change. The conceptual meaning of motivation appraisal was examined within the context of wellness motivation theory, which included an explication of the essential features of the concept meaning and dimensions across different cultural and demographic groups, as well as its relationship to other concepts within the theory (Fleury, 1991, 1993, 1996).

To construct a scale that would measure individual motivation appraisal to initiate health behavior change, the initial step in instrument development consisted of an exploratory study to identify the psychological and social processes used to initiate and sustain health behavior over time (Fleury, 1991). Qualitative data were used as a basis for analyzing and explicating the meaning of motivation appraisal as a concept central to the initiation of behavioral change, as well as to delineate a conceptual basis for instrument development (Tilden, Nelson, & May, 1990). Methods designed to preserve the meaning inherent in the qualitative data while offering a reliable and valid measurement tool consisted of procedural and interpretive processes in item generation and instrument formation (Fleury, 1993). Quantification of Index of Readiness (IR) content validity, item clarity, and homogeneity of content was established through expert ratings, following criteria established by Imle and Atwood (1988).

Initial psychometric testing of the Index of Readiness was conducted with a sample of 146 participants with diagnosed coronary artery disease (Fleury, 1994). The instrument was evaluated for reliability and validity, including internal consistency reliability and validity assessment (criterion-related validity and construct validity). Three subscales, Behavioral Reevaluation, Identification of Barriers, and Goal Commitment, were supported using exploratory factor analytic methods. Internal consistency estimates for IR subscales ranged from .72 to .86. As an estimate of criterion-related validity, concurrent validity was demonstrated through correlations between IR subscales and an Index of Current Health Behaviors (ICHB). Construct validity of the IR was estimated by examining the relationships between measures of individual health locus of control (Lau & Ware, 1981) and health value orientation (Lau, Hartman, & Ware, 1986).

Enriquez, O'Connor, and McKinsey (2000) reported preliminary data examining the relevance of the IR in predicting medication adherence in 23 males with diagnosed HIV. Participants were Caucasian ($n = 11$), African American ($n = 11$), and Hispanic ($n = 1$), with a mean age of 40 ($SD = 9.3$). Reliability estimates calculated for the three subscales Behavioral Reevaluation, Identification of Barriers, and Goal Commitment ranged from .67–.81. To determine the relationship between readiness and adherence, the three subscales were correlated with clinical indicators of adherence including CD4 counts, PCR viral load, and HIV symptoms. CD4 counts were positively and significantly correlated with Identification of Barriers ($r = .31$) and Goal Commitment ($r = .75$) at 1 month on an anti-HIV medication regimen. Correlations between CD4 count and Index of Readiness subscales ranged from .37 to .61 for patients at 2 months on an anti-HIV medication regimen. PCR viral loads were significantly, negatively correlated with Identification of Barriers ($r = -.55$) and Goal Commitment ($r = -.36$) at 1 month on an anti-HIV medication regimen. Similarly, PCR viral loads were significantly, negatively correlated with Index of Readiness subscales at 2 months on an anti-HIV medication regimen, ranging from $-.19$ to $-.52$.

Scale refinement has included evaluation of the cultural meaning and relevance of IR scale items, based on the experiences of different ethnic and demographic groups of participants attempting health behavior change (Fleury, Harrell, & Cobb, 2001). To address the lack of attention

to cultural differences in meaning and measurement of motivational predictors of health-promoting behavior, focus group methods were used
with elderly, rural-dwelling African American men and women. Focus
groups were convened at six rural community sites over a period of 2
months. Each group consisted of 6 to 10 men and women, and interviews
lasted approximately 60 minutes.

Focus group activities were guided by an open-ended response format
designed to clearly introduce the concept of motivation appraisal, evaluate the meaning and relevance of the concept and concept dimensions to
older African Americans, and explore how concept dimensions might be
operationalized in the Index of Readiness. Focus group questions specific to the concept of motivation appraisal included "What might
make you think that you need to change the ways that you take care of
yourself?," "What kinds of things make it difficult for you to take care
of yourself?," and "How do you begin to make plans to change the way
you take care of yourself?" Questions were designed to evaluate the
cultural relevance, meaning, and clarity of concept dimensions, including
Behavioral Reevaluation, Acknowledgment of Barriers, and Goal Commitment.

Focus group interviews were audiotaped and transcribed. Focus group
transcripts were reviewed to identify major themes. Data were analyzed
using a structured evaluation of the data formulated by a set of guiding
hypotheses. Data were organized into conceptual codes, with data exem-
plars to represent each of the conceptual codes. Codes were examined
for correspondence with the original concept definition and concept
dimensions. Data were compared with original Index of Readiness
measurement items to develop or adapt items that accurately reflected
informants' experience and were culturally meaningful. In item revision and the development of new items, the meaning, language, and
expression used by participants during focus group interviews were retained.

Findings from focus group interviews substantiated the meaningful-
ness of the theoretical concept of motivation appraisal among older African Americans. Data supported the inclusion of the concept dimensions
Behavioral Reevaluation and Goal Commitment, but proposed a change
in the concept of Identification of Barriers. Informants did not empha-
size specific types of barriers to behavioral change as much as the need to
create a plan for action in behavioral change. Based on this information,
a third dimension of Goal Strategies was developed. These dimensions
were individually defined, based on data generated, and as subscales,
formed the operational framework for the refinement of the Index of
Readiness. Scale items were developed or revised to correspond with data
from within each dimension of motivation appraisal. Item development
reflected readiness to initiate general health behaviors as well as items
specific to regular physical activity (Table 20.1). The revised IR consists of

9 items measuring dimensions of Behavioral Reevaluation, Goal Strategies, and Goal Commitment.

DESCRIPTION

The revised 9-item scale has a 5th grade, 1 month Flesch-Kincaid reading level. Items are formatted using a 6-point Likert scale ranging from 1 (*Strongly Disagree*), to 6 (*Strongly Agree*). The IR consists of three subscales measuring self-report: Behavioral Reevaluation, Goal Strategies, and Goal Commitment. Behavioral Reevaluation reflects the identification of a perceived discrepancy between individual behavior and the cognitive representation of individual goals and standards for behavior. Goal Strategies reflects the creation of a plan for action that facilitates the initiation of new patterns of behavior. Goal Commitment is the acceptance of responsibility to initiate and sustain health-related behavioral change. Each dimension is conceptualized as a distinct way in which individuals appraise readiness to initiate health behavior change. The scale dimensions and related items related to regular physical activity are presented in Table 20.1.

ADMINISTRATION AND SCORING

The Index of Readiness is a pencil-and-paper questionnaire and may be administered in person, by mail, or via telephone. It takes less than 10 minutes to complete. To score the instrument, item scores are summed for each subscale. Scores can range from 9 to 54. Higher scores on IR subscales indicate a greater appraisal of readiness to initiate behavioral change.

RELIABILITY AND VALIDITY EVIDENCE

Initial psychometric testing of the revised IR was conducted with a sample of 83 rural-dwelling African Americans with a mean age of 75 ($SD = 7.8$, range: 60–98 years). The majority of participants were female (87%), had less than a high school education (68%), were retired (88%), and were single as a result of widowhood (80%).

Estimates of the internal consistency of the scale were calculated for each of the three subscales of the revised IR. Subscale alpha reliability ranged from .74 to .89. Item-to-total correlations ranged from .40 to .76. Item-to-item correlations had greater than 70% above .30, with the majority between .33 and .69. Mean score for Behavioral Reevaluation was 11.6 ($SD = 2.34$), Goal Strategy was 11.1 ($SD = 2.61$), and Goal Commitment was 12.1 ($SD = 2.21$). Construct validity of the instrument was examined

TABLE 20.1 Dimensions of Appraisal of Readiness

Subscale Dimensions/Definition	Scale Items Specific to Physical Activity
Behavioral reevaluation Identification of value/behavior incongruence which directs the formation. of relevant goals in behavioral change.	I think about what might happen if I don't begin a program of physical activity.
	I don't participate in physical activity as often as I feel that I could.
	I think that I need to change some of the things that keep me from staying physically active.
Goal strategies Creation of an individual plan for action which facilitates the initiation of new patterns of behavior.	I have thought about ways I can make physical activity fit into my life.
	I have planned new ways to stay physically active.
	I have a plan for how to overcome barriers to physical activity.
Goal commitment Individual acceptance of responsibility to initiate and sustain health behavior change.	I am willing to make sacrifices in order to be physically active on a regular basis.
	I am determined to succeed in making physical activity part of my life.
	I am committed to making lasting changes in the ways that I stay physically active.

through path analysis correlating IR subscales with theoretically related constructs of self-regulation and the performance of regular physical activity (Fleury, Belyea, & Harrell, 2000). The motivation appraisal variable Goal Commitment was significantly related to the self-regulation variables cognitive restructuring, stimulus control and behavioral monitoring, emphasizing the importance of commitment in the ongoing regulation of behavioral change. The variable Behavioral Reevaluation was significantly related to physical activity measured as estimated weekly metabolic equivalent minutes.

Thomas and colleagues (Thomas, Hilsabeck, Carlson, Hassanein, & Perry, 2001) explored readiness to change health behaviors in 109 patients (66% male) with chronic hepatitis C. Mean age was 45.5 (*SD* =7.02), years of education was 13.47 (*SD* =2.29). An exploratory factor analysis using orthogonal rotation supported the 3-factor structure, Behavioral Reevaluation, Goal Strategies, and Goal Commitment, accounting for 72.8% of the variance. Internal consistency reliability for the total scale was .79. Construct validity was demonstrated through correlations between IR subscales and theoretically related criterion measures. In general, the Behavioral Reevaluation subscale correlated significantly with measures of mental health and self-efficacy (ranging from −.29 to −.39). The Goal Strategies subscale correlated significantly with measures of motivation for change (r = .45 to .60); the Goal Commitment subscale correlated significantly with physical symptoms and associated distress (r = .27 to .36). There was a significant gender difference, with females indicating greater readiness to change health behaviors.

Whittemore (2000) evaluated the efficacy of the Index of Readiness in exploring the process of integrating lifestyle changes related to noninsulin-dependent diabetes mellitus treatment recommendations and glycemic control. Using a multimethod design that included interpretive methods, Whittemore substantiated the relevance of the IR related to health-promoting behaviors and glycemic control of individuals with NIDDM. Interpretive methods supported the relevance and importance of the concept of motivation appraisal in the experience of integration and lifestyle change in NIDDM.

CONCLUSIONS AND RECOMMENDATIONS

The creation of measurement scales that reflect individual and cultural meaning challenges researchers to continue to devise more effective ways or representing and investigating the complexities of motivation in behavioral change. Continued exploration and ongoing methodologic efforts are needed both to test the relevance of existing measurement instruments and to explore the meaning of motivational concepts across cultural and demographic groups.

Findings presented indicate that initial efforts in the development, refinement, and psychometric testing of the IR have been successful. The measure is both reliable and valid and is sensitive both to the magnitude of individual appraisal of readiness to create behavioral change and to variations in appraisal of readiness during preparation for behavioral change. The IR provides a basis for individualized education and intervention strategies that support health-promoting behaviors. Continued testing and refinement of the IR will allow further exploration of the processes inherent in health behavior change as well as the development of interventions designed to enhance motivation in risk factor modification efforts.

REFERENCES

Bandura, A. (1986). *Social foundations of thought and action: A social cognitive theory.* Englewood Cliffs, NJ: Prentice-Hall.

Bandura, A. (1989). Regulation of cognitive processes through perceived self-efficacy. *Developmental Psychology, 25,* 729–735.

Carver, C. S., & Scheier, M. F. (1981). *Attention and self-regulation: A control theory approach to human behavior.* New York: Springer-Verlag.

D'Andrade, R. G. (1990). Some propositions about the relations between culture and human cognition. In: J. W. Stigler, R. A. Shweder, & G. Herdt, (Eds.), *Culture psychology: Essays on comparative human development* (pp. 65–129). Cambridge, MA: Cambridge University Press.

Enriquez, M., O'Connor, M., & McKinsey, D. (2000). *A pilot study to examine a multidisciplinary intervention to increase adherence to anti-HIV medications in patients previously failing therapy.* Unpublished manuscript.

Ewart, C. (1991). Social action theory for a public health psychology. *American Psychologist, 9,* 931–946.

Fleury, J. (1991). The qualitative generation of wellness motivation theory. *Nursing Research, 40,* 286–291.

Fleury, J. (1993). The challenge of preserving qualitative meaning in instrument development. *Journal of Nursing Measurement, 3,* 135–144.

Fleury, J. (1994). The index of readiness: Development and psychometric analysis. *Journal of Nursing Measurement, 2,* 143–154.

Fleury, J. (1996). Theoretical relevance of wellness motivation theory. *Nursing Research, 45,* 277–283.

Fleury, J., Belyea, M., & Harrell, J. (2000). Physical activity among elderly African Americans: A test of the wellness motivation theory. *Annals of Behavioral Medicine, 22* (2000 Suppl.), S119.

Fleury, J., Harrell, J., & Cobb, B (2001). Regular physical activity in older African Americans. In: S. G. Funk, E. M. Tornquist, J. Leeman, M. S. Miles, & J. S. Harrell (Eds). *Key aspects of preventing and managing chronic illness.* (pp. 84–94). New York: Springer Publishing Co.

Gollwitzer, P. M. (1987). *Motivation, intention and volition.* New York: Springer-Verlag.

Imle, M., & Atwood, J. (1988). Retaining qualitative validity while gaining quantitative reliability and validity: Development of the transition to parenthood concerns scale. *Advances in Nursing Science, 11,* 61–75.

Karoly, P. (1995). Self-control theory. In: W. O'Donohue, & L. Krasner (Eds.) *Theories of behavior therapy* (pp. 259–286.). Washington, DC: American Psychological Association.

Kuhl, J. (1987). Action control: The maintenance of motivational states. In F. Halisch & J. Kuhl (Eds.). *Motivation, intention and volition* (pp. 279–292). New York: Springer-Verlag.

Lau, R. R., Hartman, K. A., & Ware, J. F. (1986). Health as a value: Methodological and theoretical considerations. *Health Psychology, 5,* 25–43.

Lau, R. R., & Ware, J. F. (1981). Refinements in the measure of health-specific locus of control beliefs. *Medical Care, 19,* 1147–1156.

Markus, H., & Nurius, P. (1986). Possible selves. *American Psychologist, 41,* 954–969.

Markus, H., & Wurf, E. (1987). The dynamic self-concept: A social psychological perspective. *Annual Review of Psychology, 38,* 299–337.

Nuttin, J. R. (1987). The respective roles of cognition and motivation in behavioral dynamics, Intention, and volition. In: F. Halisch, J. Kuhl (Eds.), *Motivation, intention and volition* (pp. 309–320). New York: Springer-Verlag.

Public Health Service, U. S. Department of Health and Human Services. (1990). *Healthy people: National health promotion and disease prevention objectives.* Washington, DC: U.S. Government Printing Office.

Thomas, J. L., Hilsabeck, R. C., Carlson, M. D., Hassinein, T. I., & Perry, W. (2001). Validation of the Index of Readiness Scale in patients with chronic hepatitis C. *Annals of Behavioral Medicine, 23,* S187.

Tilden, V. P., Nelson, C. A., & May, B. A. (1990). The IPRI inventory: Development and psychometric characteristics. *Nursing Research, 39,* 337–343.

Whittemore, R. (2000). *A coaching intervention to integrate lifestyle change in adults with non-insulin dependent diabetes mellitus.* Unpublished Doctoral dissertation, Boston College School of Nursing, Boston.

APPENDIX: INDEX OF READINESS—GENERAL ITEMS

Directions: These questions reflect how people feel about the ways they try to stay healthy. Please answer each statement by first thinking about the statement, and then circling the response which best describes the extent to which you agree or disagree with the statement.

Response Choices:
1 = Strongly Disagree
2 = Moderately Disagree
3 = Disagree
4 = Agree
5 = Moderately Agree
6 = Strongly Agree

1. I think about what might happen if I don't change the ways I take care of myself.　　　1 2 3 4 5 6

2. I don't take care of myself as well as I feel that I could.　　　1 2 3 4 5 6

3. I think that I need to change some of the ways that I take care of myself.　　　1 2 3 4 5 6

4. I have planned new ways to change how I take care of myself.　　　1 2 3 4 5 6

5. I have thought about how to make changing the ways I take care of myself fit into my life.　　　1 2 3 4 5 6

6. I have a plan for how to overcome barriers to changing the ways I take care of myself.　　　1 2 3 4 5 6

7. I am willing to make sacrifices in order to change the ways that I take care of myself.　　　1 2 3 4 5 6

8. I am determined to succeed in changing the ways that I take care of myself.　　　1 2 3 4 5 6

9. I am committed to making lasting changes in the ways that I take care of myself.　　　1 2 3 4 5 6

Index